THE

CHIROPRACTOR

(1914)

Contents: The Moral and Religious Duty of a Chiropractor; Chiropractic a Science, an Art and the Philosophy Thereof; Nerve Vibration; Inflammation; Vertebral Luxations; Health, Disease, Life and Death; Rickets; Biology; Function; Vertebral Adjusting; The Nervous System; Neuritis, Arteritis and Rheumatism; Fever; Constipation; Trauma, Toxine and Auto-Suggestion; Catarrh; Impulse; The Normal and Abnormal Movements of the Vertebral Column; Spinal Pathogenesis; Palpation and Nerve Tracing; Bones and Nerves; Pyorrhea Alveolaris.

D.D. Palmer

ISBN 1-56459-775-X

Kessinger Publishing's Rare Reprints
Thousands of Scarce and Hard-to-Find Books!

. . .
. . .
. . .
. . .
. . .
. . .
. . .
. . .
. . .
. . .
. . .
. . .
. . .
. . .
. . .
. . .
. . .
. . .
. . .
. . .

We kindly invite you to view our extensive catalog list at:
http://www.kessinger.net

Warning—Disclaimer

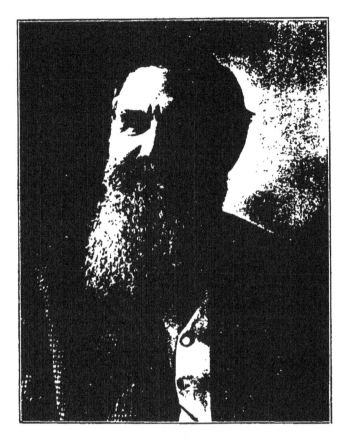

D. D. Palmer.

Founder of Chiropractic. The Creator of Chiropractic Science. The Originator of
Vertebral Adjusting. The Developer of Chiropractic Philosophy. The Foun-
tain Head of the Principles of Chiropractic, their skillful application
for the use of humanity and the reasons why and how they
Govern Life in Health and Disease. Lecturer and
Demonstrator on the Science, Art and
Philosophy of Chiropractic.

CONTENTS:

The Moral and Religious Duty of a Chiropractor.

The following has been sharply criticised by a few chiropractors, but not as severely, nor by as many as was my announcement of the moving of joints by hand. A part of this criticism was based upon rival jealousy, the balance because of wrong impressions. That which was on account of a lack of information discontinued as soon as the would-be critics were well informed. I have received greater applause at the close of the following lecture from my classes than from any other. Every important chiropractic idea that I have advanced has been bitterly assailed, yet, although somewhat discouraged at times, I have not turned from that which I knew was correct.

The Constitution of the United States declares that "Congress shall make no law respecting an established religion, or prohibiting the free exercise thereof." The great state of California has granted the same privilege in its medical act, by declaring in Sec. 17, "Nor shall this act be construed so as to discriminate against . . . the practice of religion." It was quite mindful and generous of those who framed the California Medical Act to coincide with the Constitution of the United States in not allowing the Medical Act to conflict with the Constitution of the United States nor interfere with the religious duty of chiropractors, a privilege already conferred upon them. It now becomes us as chiropractors to assert our religious rights.

There could be no religion without science and philosophy.

Other states than California, in their laws to regulate the practice of medicine, have been mindful of religious conscience.

Kansas. "Nothing in this act shall be construed as interfering with any religious beliefs in the treatment of disease."

Virginia. "This act does not . . . interfere in any way with the practice of religion."

Washington. "This act does not apply to . . . nor interfere in anyway with the practice of religion."

Illinois. "Nothing in this act applies to . . . any person who administers to or treats the sick or suffering by mental or spiritual means without the use of any drug or material remedy."

The new law of 1913 of the state of California says, "Nor shall this act be construed so as to discriminate against . . . the practice of religion."

Chiropractic is a science and an art. The philosophy of chiropractic consists of the reasons given for the principles which compose the science and the movements which have to do with the art.

1

Science is accepted, accumulated knowledge, systematized and formulated with reference to the existence of general facts—the operation of general laws concerning one subject. Chiropractic is the name of a classified, indexed, knowledge of successive sense impressions of biology—the science of life—which science I created out of principles which have existed as long as the vertebrata.

Science is the knowledge of knowing. Scientific religion embraces a systematic knowledge of facts which can be verified by conscious cerebration. Knowledge is superior to faith and belief. Faith is an inward acceptance of some personal act; we believe thon is trustworthy, therefore, we have faith. Faith is a union of belief and trust. Belief is an intellectual process, the acceptance of some thing as true on other grounds than personal observation and experience. Faith implies a trust in a person. We may believe in a proposition in which no person is implied or thought of. Knowledge is knowing, we know from personal evidence. That which may be evidence to you may not be to me. That which we may accept as evidence today may not appeal to us as such tomorrow. Our belief, faith and knowledge depend upon our education. Our education depends upon our environments. Art relates to something to be done. Chiropractic art consists in the aptitude of adjusting displaced vertebrae, of which art I am the originator.

Chiropractic philosophy is the knowledge of the phenomena of life, as explained by the understanding of the principles, of the science and art. In my work on the Science, Art and Philosophy of Chiropractic I have given an extensive explanation of the laws of life and the nature of disease.

The practice of chiropractic includes a moral obligation and a religious duty. To comprehend these responsibilities it is absolutely necessary that the chiropractor should be able to understand and define chiropractic science. He must know not only the basic principle upon which it is founded and the constitutional parts which form its scientific structure, but, also, the philosophy of the science and art of vertebral adjusting. To absorb and digest these all important and essential ideas and make them a part of one's very being, requires a close study of The Chiropractor's Adjuster.

Chiropractic deals with biology. It is the only comprehensive system which answers the time-worn question "what is life."

Scientific chiropractors are versed in the principles of chiropractic. They live according to its rules. They philosophize on the art of relieving abnormal conditions by adjusting displaced bones. As Educated Intelligences, they relieve undue pressure on nerves in order that Innate may transmit and receive impulses to and from the various parts of the body in a normal manner. They desire to understand the nature of our physical existence and assign natural causes for both normal and abnormal functions.

As a science chiropractic explains local and general death to be but the result of law, a step on the road of eternal progression; that any deviation from tone, the basis of chiropractic, is disease.

As a philosophy it is the science of all sciences. It deals with subjective, ethical religion—the science which treats of the existence, character and attributes of God, the All-pervading Universal Intelligence. Its possibilities will become unlimited, when His laws and our duties as a segmented, personified, portion thereof, are scientifically understood. It will lessen disease, poverty and crime, empty our jails, penitentiaries and insane asylums and assist us to prepare for the existence beyond the transition called death. It explains why all persons are not equal, mentally and physically; or, if born alike, why some become superior or inferior to others similarly situated, why certain individuals are not able to express themselves as intelligently as others, why some persons are not mentally and physically alike at all times. To make clear this difference I will give a case and its termination under chiropractic adjusting. Ed., seventeen years of age, was hemiplegic in the left half of his body since birth. He had not uttered a word that was understood by his parents or friends. Mentally he was that of a child three years of age. Six weeks of chiropractic adjusting caused the distorted sixth dorsal articulation to become normal in shape and to occupy its normal position, releasing a stretched condition on the sixth pair of dorsal nerves, creating a normal tension of nerves and muscles, the usual force to impulses, arousing the normal amount of energy, consequently, the normal expression of ideas. In six weeks Ed's mentality and language was that of others of like age and environments. Conation (desire and volition)was equal to those of cognition and feeling. He became subject to the law of duty, capable of acting through his moral sense of right—he was a moral agent. He was, alike, intellectual in each of the three great divisions of the mind. I had performed a moral duty, as well as a religious duty. It points out the conditions upon which both health and disease depend. It explains why and how one person becomes affected with disease while his associate or neighobr, apparently living under the same conditions, remains well. Furthermore, it makes plain the reason why one, or more, of the bodily functions are performed in an excessive or in a deficient degree of frequency or intensity, either of which condition is a form of disease.

When Educated and Innate Intelligences are able to converse with each other, (a possibility which not a very distant future may disclose), we shall be able to make a correct diagnosis. Heretofore, these two intelligences have misunderstood each other concerning the laws which govern life. When the science of biology is correctly understood the span of life will be more than doubled.

Chiropractic has pulled aside the curtain of ignorance which obscured the cause of disease; in time it will lift the veil of superstition, which has obstructed our vision of the great beyond. In time, spiritual existence will be as well known and comprehended as that of the physical world.

Chiropractic science includes biology—the science of life—in this world, and the recognition of a spiritual existence in the next. The principles which compose it are substantive in their independence and incentive to human and spiritual progress. They originate in Divinity, the Universal Intelligence, and constitute the essential qualities of life which, having begun in this world, are never ending.

It is an educational, scientific, religious system. It associates its practice, belief and knowledge with that of religion. It imparts instruction relating both to this world and the one to come. Supreme spiritual existence can only be obtained through earthly experience. Chiropractic sheds enlightenment upon physical life and spiritual existence, the latter being only a continuation of the former.

Chiropractic literature makes use of such technical terms as are calculated to enlighten mankind in regard to the Universal Intelligence which the Christian world has seen fit to acknowledge as God. It enables its disciples to recognize the above facts, and teaches them how to adjust their lives accordingly.

The casual thinker is obliged to admit that the universe is composed of intelligence and matter; that the latter is neither intelligent nor creative, while the former is omnipresent, filling all space; that this creative intelligence uses material substance for expression, and that life is the direct result of this intelligence seeking advancement toward perfection by the use of visible, corporeal organisms.

Man is a dual entity, composed of intelligence and matter, spirit and material, the immortal and mortal, the everlasting and the transient. The manifestation of such an existence is intelligent action.

Chiropractors, especially, are aiding in this great advancement by adjusting the osseous structure, the position of which has to do with determining normal and abnormal tension, for in whatever part function is abnormally performed tonicity is either lacking or excessive—Creative Intelligence is prevented from expressing itself normally. Many a child has been injured at birth by a vertebral displacement which caused an impingement upon one or more of the spinal nerves, as they emanate from the spinal canal, the fibers of which are distributed to certain organs. The result of this excessive tension is physical or mental debility, often both, which, from a lack of pathological knowledge, may be lifelong; the mental defect extending even into the next world. For we retain only that which has been acquired during this earthly, preparatory existence. By properly adjusting the neuroskeleton, these unfortunates may be enabled to acquire sufficient knowledge, rightfully due them, to become useful members of society and enjoy life in this world and the one to come. The chiropractor who can accomplish the above desirable results and refuses to do so, as a religious duty, should be compelled to perform it as a moral obligation.

Frank, a young man, twenty-one years of age, was brought to me for correction. Physically, he was a cripple in upper and lower limbs. His case was considered one of cerebral disease, an imbecile. An M. D. would say, his diseased condition was congenital, acquired at the moment of birth, but, to a chiropractor it was acquired; in fact, all diseases are acquired, have their causes, whether before or after birth. In this case it was because of the sixth dorsal vertebra being displaced at birth. By daily adjusting the vertebra which had become abnormally shaped, was grown to the normal and placed in the usual position, thereby enabling the spirit to perform its desired avocation of creating a normal physical and the accumulating of normal ideas which will last throughout eternity. By so doing I was performing a service, a duty, I assumed when I accepted the trust bestowed upon me. By so doing I was not only performing a normal obligation, but, also, a (subjective) religious duty.

I hold it to be self-evident that all men and women who have acquired sufficient knowledge and skill to remove the nerve tension which prevents physical, mental and spiritual development, are engaged in a work of a higher order than that ordinarily required of, and performed by, the physician. They are practically the moral duties, and obligations of religion and any attempt to prevent such acts by law is an unmitigated crime against humanity.

Chiropractic science, its art and philosophy, deal with human and spiritual phenomena. The conscientious reverent acknowledgement of the phenomena, in sentiment and act, connects the spiritual with the physical, and constitutes in its fullest and highest sense a religion.

The knowledge and philosophy given me by Dr. Jim Atkinson, an intelligent spiritual being, together with explanations of phenomena, principles resolved from causes, effects, powers, laws and utility, appealed to my reason.

The method by which I obtained an explanation of certain physical phenomena, from an intelligence in the spiritual world, is known in biblical language as inspiration. In a great measure The Chiropractor's Adjuster was written under such spiritual promptings.

The object of a chiropractic education is the attainment of information concerning the origin, development, structure, and functions of our physical organism, the phenomena of physical earth-life and that of spiritual existence. These are acquired by observation and demonstration. Chiropractors declare that God is the All-pervading Intelligence, that each individual, segmented portion of spirit is a part of that intelligent creative principle; that only matter changes its form; that spirit modifies its environment, and dissolution is but a process of reproduction. Chiropractic science elucidates the problems of life, gives us the incentive to human endeavor and the agency by which sin, the violation, willfully or accidentally, of moral or natural laws, may be eradicated by appropriate adjustment of the neuroskeleton.

The cumulative function pertains to intellectual growth, whether sane or insane. As we retain our mentalities and carry with us to the great beyond only that which we mentally gather, it is necessary, in fact, it is a religious duty, to so care for our physical beings that our intellectual attainment may be of the very best.

The philosophy of chiropractic teaches the Universality of Intelligence and that its aim is always onward and upward toward perfection. This truth makes the practice of chiropractic a moral and a religious duty both in theory and in fact.

Religion may be objective in its character. As a cult it consists of the rites and ceremonies pertaining to the worship of a Deity, and only known by external, devotional acts of reverence. Subjective religion includes the moral and religious duty, the inner intellectual feeling, the science which treats of the existence, character and attributes of God and His laws regarding our duty toward Him. The former is that of theology; it includes the peculiar modes of divine worship which belong to and make the special distinction of tribes, nations and communities. The latter is ethical religion and deals only with positives, existing phenomena, properties which are knowable, together with their invariable relations of co-existence and succession. A belief in magic, the assistance of secret forces in nature, constitutes the essential of objective religion. The supernormal, the mysterious potency hidden from the understanding, the supernatural, the occult secret power, is the original, the basic element, the morbid outgrowth of subjective religion. Chiropractors deal only with moral obligations and subjective, ethical religion.

I do not propose to change chiropractic, either in its science, art or philosophy, into a religion. The moral and religious duty of a chiropractor are not synonomous with the science, art and philosophy of chiropractic. There is a vast difference between a theological religion and a religious duty; between the precepts and practices of religion and that of chiropractic. A person may be a conscientious devotee of any theological creed and yet be a strict, upright, exalted principled practitioner of chiropractic.

Chiro Religio, Chiropractic Religion, the Religion of Chiropractic and the Religious Duty of a Chiropractor are one and the same.

Willard Carver, D. C., asks, "Do you believe it wise to denominate chiropractic as a religion?" This question is equal to asking a physician, Do you believe it wise to denominate medicine (not the practice) as a religion?

Webster's Dictionary, latest edition, date 1910, gives near the bottom of page 1801, fifth column, the Latin phrase, religio medici, meaning, a physician's religion. Has not a chiropractor as much right to a religion as a practitioner of medicine? Is not chiro religio as consistent and comprehensible as religio medici?

"Do you believe it wise to denominate chiropractic as a religion?"

To denominate is to name, designate, specify or characterize. Wherein have I expressed a desire to RE-name the science, art and philosophy of chiropractic? In what sentence have I designated chiropractic by any other distinctive title than that by which it is now known? In what paragraph have I specified or characterized chiropractic as a religion? The science, art and philosophy of chiropractic is one thing: the moral and religious duty of a chiropractor is a different proposition. The founder, the fountain head, the creator, the originator, the developer, the one who named the science, art and philosophy of vertebral adjusting, says emphatically, it is not wise to denominate chiropractic by any other name or title than the one by which it is known the world over.

F. W. Carlin, D. C., writes me, "The Religion of Chiropractic is absurd."

I fully agree with Dr. Carlin. To say or think that the science, the art, or the philosophy of chiropractic, or that chiropractic, the three combined, has a religion, is really absurd and ridiculous.

He also says, "All religions are more or less based upon superstition. There is nothing superstitious about chiropractic."

He is right. All methods of treating diseases, as well as all forms of religion, are based upon superstition. Chiropractic as a science, as an art and the philosophy thereof, also, the moral and religious duty of chiropractors, are free of superstition, they are based upon the knowledge of principles and facts.

There is the moral and religious science of chiropractic, the moral and religious philosophy of chiropractic, the moral and religious responsibility attached to the practice of chiropractic, the moral and religious liberty granted to chiropractors by the Constitution of the United States; also, the moral theology of chiropractic, known in the California Medical Act as religion.

Morally, chiropractors are in duty bound to help humanity physically. Religiously, they are required to render spiritual service toward God, the Universal Intelligence, by relieving mankind of their fetters, adjusting the tension-frame of the nervous system, the physical lines of communication to and from the spirit. By so doing they greatly aid intellectual attainment and progress toward perfection through the untrammeled, mental reception of intelligent expressions of individual spirits. By correcting the skeletal frame the spirit is permitted to assume normal control, and produce normal expression.

The importance of bone-pressure on nerves as a disease producer (violation of public or divine law, the result of morbid conditions), is receiving attention by physicians.

The Los Angeles Times of May 25, 1911, gives a case of kleptomania wherein the knife was used to remove bone-pressure on nerves which were supposed to cause "criminal propensities." The "pretty 22-year-old woman, an uncontrollable kleptomaniac, had served one year in prison for shoplifting." The physicians considered her case "one of disease rather than of crime."

A month after the operation "a thorough revolution had taken place in her mental faculties. Her change for the good is going to be just as strongly pronounced as was her bent for the bad."

PASADENA, March 30.—Mrs. Jean Thurner of No. 315 West Avenue

50, Los Angeles, who attained almost world-wide fame two years ago when she underwent an operation for kleptomania at the American Hospital in Berkeley, at the hands of Dr. Herbert Rowell, who removed a piece of skull as large as a dollar from the top of the head, on the right side, was arrested at her home yesterday morning at the instigation of Detective Charles Betts, charged with the theft of diamonds and rings valued at $581 from three Pasadena jewelry stores.

Instead of using the knife and drugs, chiropractors substitute hand-adjustment of the displaced portion of the neuroskeleton which presses upon or against some portion of the nervous system, which injures, instead of protecting, the filamentous bands of nervous tissue that connect the parts of the nervous system with each other and transmit impulses to the various organs of the body.

The principles which form chiropractic science have always existed; and are now being revealed to the world by D. D. Palmer, through the Chiropractor's Adjuster. This revelation of the science, art and philosophy was given by one who tells me that he is indebted to those who are farther advanced in the knowledge of physical and spiritual phenomena than he is.

Through and by these discoveries chiropractors are able to relieve diseases which heretofore were pronounced by the medical profession as incurable. Thousands of cases of this kind can be cited.

I created a science out of the principles revealed to me and named it chiropractic. I correlated the art of adjusting displaced vertebrae together with the philosophy of the science and art. That these revelations were not made along the lines of medical and theological investigations is not strange when we consider that very few great discoveries have been made by those who were expecting results in certain smoothly worn grooves of stereotyped education. It is not surprising that those who have given to the world its greatest and grandest thoughts have been, more or less, connected with those who had passed into the spiritual existence.

Chiropractic gives relief to, and opens up a haven for, those who are ailing, making them physically, mentally and spiritually invigorated and whole. This noble work results in the direct salvation of countless numbers of mental and physical wrecks; for, the consequences of their disabilities do not stop at the grave, but continue on and on into the eternal spiritual existence.

An author on chiropractic states: "The special philosophy which he has worked out assigned as the foundation."

Philosophy, special or general, is not the foundation upon which I built the science of chiropractic. Its science is based on tone. Tone is the standard from which we note the variations of structure, temperature, tonicity, elasticity, renitency and tension; it is the standard of health; any deviation therefrom is disease. Tone is the BASIC PRINCIPLE, the one from which all other principles, which compose the science, have sprung.

Chiropractic is a science. The art of adjusting is the systematic, skillful application of chiropractic principles. Much study and correct reasoning upon the laws which constitute this science have developed its philosophy. The foundation of chiropractic does not consist of its philosophy, nor of the art of adjusting. I discovered the principles of which chiropractic science is constituted. By skill, directed by the knowledge of the science and its philosophy, I originated the art of adjusting. A knowledge of the science, art and philosophy of chiropractic contain a moral and a religious duty; morally, it serves as our basis of humane action according to our reason and judgment concerning our physical welfare; religiously, it governs our motives of divine duty with respect to the advancement of our spiritual existence throughout eternity. Its principles embrace the faith, belief, practice, obligations and conduct of our lives toward God and man.

Those who have a knowledge of, or a belief in, a future state of existence, regardless of church or creed, can become believers in and practitioners of, the religion OF chiropractors.

That which I named Innate (born with) is a segment of that Intelligence which fills the universe. This universal, All Wise, is metamerized, divided into metameres as needed by each individualized being. This somatome of the whole never sleeps, nor tires, recognizes neither darkness or distance, is not subject to material laws, bodily wants are not essential, substantial conditions are not needed for its existence. It continues to care for and direct the organic functions of the body as long as the soul holds body and spirit together.

Physicians deal with the physical only; chiropractors with both the physical and the spiritual.

Psycological investigation reveals the fact that the spirit of man is a part of the All Wise Spirit, the Great Creator, and as such possesses in an infinitesimal degree all the potentialities of omniscience and omnipotence existing in God, just as one drop of the ocean contains, in minature, all the qualities of the briny deep as a whole.

There are those who think the spirit of man has an abiding place in the solar plexus, or in the spinal column, or in the medulla oblongata, or in the cerebellum, or in the cerebrum, or at least in some portion of the encephalon, but just what part or how much space occupied has not been determined.

The spirit holds the same relation to the body as God, the All Wise Intelligence does to the Universe. If you can locate the one, you can designate the location and define the limits of the other. God is indwelling in the universe, everywhere present; He occupies every part thereof; likewise, the spirit permeates every portion of the body in which it dwells. God does not depend upon the universe for His existence, neither does the spirit rely upon the body for its continued manifestations.

Although the surgeon cannot locate or dissect the spirit, that which creates intelligent action, yet we are conscious of this vital entity.

Knowledge of, or a belief in, the continuity of life has a tendency to uplift humanity, to make of man a desirable neighbor, a good citizen, a moral upright being and a practical understanding of right and wrong.

Innate is embodied as a personified part of Universal Intelligence, therefore, co-eternal with the all-creative force. This indwelling portion of the Eternal is in our care for improvement. The intellectual expansion of Innate is in proportion to the normal transmission of impulses over the nervous system; for this reason the body functions should be kept in the condition of tone. Communication with the Eternal Spirit, the Creator, is the goal of all religions.

There is no living religion without a doctrine; a doctrine, however elaborate, does not constitute a religion. The doctrine of our principles, faith and knowledge, are as follows:

I believe, in fact know, that the universe consists of Intelligence and Matter. This intelligence is known to the Christian world as God. As a spiritual intelligence it finds expression through the animal and vegetable creation, man being the highest manifestation. I believe that this Intelligence is segmented into as many parts as there are individual expressions of life; that spirit, whether considered as a whole or individually, is advancing upward and onward toward perfection; that in all animated nature this Intelligence is expressed through the nervous system, which is the means of communication to and from individualized spirit; that the condition known as TONE is the tension and firmness, the renitency and elasticity of tissue in a state of health, normal existence; that the mental and physical condition known as disease is a disordered state because of an unusual amount of tension above or below that of tone; that normal and abnormal amounts of strain or laxity are due to the position of the osseous framework, the neuroskeleton, which not only serves as a protector to the nervous system, but, also, as a regulator of tension; that Universal Intelligence, the Spirit as a whole or in its segmented parts, is eternal in its existence; that physiological disintegration and somatic death are changes of the material only; that the present and future make-up of individualized spirits depend upon the cumulative mental function which, like all other functions, is modified by the structural condition of the impulsive, transmitting, nervous system; that criminality is but the result of abnormal nervous tension; that our individualized, segmented spiritual entities carry with them into the future spiritual state that which has been mentally accumulated during our physical existence; that spiritual existence, like the physical, is progressive; that a correct understanding of these principles and the practice of them constitute the religion of chiropractic; that the existence and personal identity of individualized intelligences continue after the change known as death; that life in this world and the next is continuous—one of eternal progression.

"There is a natural body, and there is a spiritual body." 1 Cor. iv:44.

The spiritual and the physical are counterparts of each other, duplicates in form, shape, size and color. The evidence given by seers of every nation in all ages has been that a likeness exists between the creator and the created.

Locating the spirit in the brain, the encephalon, the mass of nervous matter contained within the brain-case, is circumscribed and yet not definite. The nervous mass within the cranium includes the two hemispheres of the cerebrum, the three divisions of the cerebellum, the pons varolii and medulla oblongata. Morphologically, these seven divisions of the encephalon are derived from the fore brain, the mid brain, the hind brain and the end brain.

The muscular, vascular and nervous systems permeate every avenue throughout the body. The conscious, characteristic actions of personified intelligence are performed through the nervous filaments of the body in which the spirit tabernacles.

The spiritual intelligence controls unintelligent matter through the nervous system. Each and every portion of the body is permeated by the spirit and its means of communication.

All functional acts are performed by the involuntary nerves; they direct organic life. The voluntary are those under the control of the human will, they look after the environments, that which supports and constitutes animal life.

There are two series of ganglia (nerve centers) lying along each side and to the front of the vertebral column, reaching from the occiput to the coccyx, fibers of which extend into the cranial, the thoracic, the abdominal and the pelvic cavities; these communicating nerve branches connect the vertebral chains to the various organs, vessels and viscera.

There are 144, or more, nerve centers, sympathetic nerve ganglia, designated by physiologists as so many brains differing in size, color, texture, functions, location, and more especially in the impulses received and distributed.

The controlling intelligence is everywhere present, manifesting through the nervous system its desires for advancement, making use of these nerve centers as receiving and distributing stations.

The founder of chiropractic has located the spirit in man, found its abiding place to be throughout the entire body, a position from which each and every nerve ganglia may be used for receiving and forwarding impulses.

Therefore, inasmuch as the light of life was revealed to me in order that I should enlighten the world, and as our physical health and the intellectual progress of the personified portion of the Universal Intelligence depend upon the proper alignment of the skeletal frame, I feel it my right and bounden duty to replace any displaced portion thereof, so that our physical and spiritual faculties may be fully and normally expressed, thereby not only enhancing our present condition, but making ourselves the better prepared to enter the next stage of existence to which this earthly existence is but a preliminary, a preparatory step.

By correcting these displacements of osseous tissue, the tension frame of the nervous system, I claim that I am rendering obedience, adoration and honor to the All-Wise Spiritual Intelligence, as well as a service to the segmented, individual portions thereof—a duty I owe to both God and mankind. In accordance with this aim and end, the Constitution of the United States and the statutes personal of California confer upon me and all persons of chiropractic faith the inalienable right to practice our religion without restraint or hindrance.

Chiropractic a Science, an Art and the Philosophy Thereof.

It has been said that science is a stranger to and nowise accounts for the peculiar contents of the book of life.

Medical men have never been able to harmonize the science of medicine with organic functions in health and disease.

Science is the registered mental account of our surroundings; it is common sense—we desire to know things as they are.

Chiropractic embraces the science of life, the knowledge of how organisms act in health and disease, also the art of adjusting the neuro-skeleton.

An organism is an organized body, such is known as the living economy, the regulation of the parts of an organic whole, the aggregate of the parts and laws governing an organism. Ecology, or bionomics, is that branch of biology which deals with the mutual relations between organisms and their environment, the effect which our surroundings has upon life, the modification of vital actions which are directed by an intelligence. Bionomic forces are those external forces, other than vital forces, which influence the changes incident to the development of life. Bionomy is the laws of life; the science which treats of laws regulating the vital functions. Biologas is the living and intelligent power displayed in organic activities. Bionergy is the life-force, the force exercised in living organisms. An organism is any individual animal or plant. Any living being is an organism. The collective parts which compose an organized body, together with the laws which govern their action constitutes an organism. An individual so constituted that it may carry on the activities of life by means of its organs, which, although differing in function, yet are mutually dependent upon each other for their individual acts is an organism. An organized body endowed with a separate existence, whose vital acts depend upon the aggregation of organs, constitutes an organism.

The science of chiropractic has lead to the creation of the art of vertebral adjusting.

The philosophy of chiropractic (the science and the art) consists of the reasons for the principles which have lead up to and the wherefore of vertebral adjusting.

Science refers to that which is to be known; art to that which is to be done; philosophy gives the reasons why of the method and the way in which it is to be performed.

A science is composed of principles which coincide with mental and physical facts. I have systematized the principles of biology, thereby

13

creating a science. The theory of chiropractic embraces the speculative principles upon which the art of vertebral adjusting is based. The study of chiropractic includes the consideration of the three divisions, viz., the science, art and the philosophy of the two just mentioned.

Chiropractic to be a science must be specific. In order to be scientific it must contain the knowledge of the principles and facts of biology reduced to an unvarying law and embodied into a system. Where science ends faith begins.

To know the science of chiropractic is to have a knowledge of the principles which compose it. The ability to put that knowledge into practice is chiropractic art.

Knowledge embraces all that we know from whatever source derived or obtained, or by whatever process acquired; it is the aggregate of facts, truths and principles obtained and retained by the mind or spirit through reason, objective perception, derived from the use of the external senses, or of intuition, subjective immediate knowing of the inner animating intelligence.

Beyond the region of knowledge is that of nescience, lack of knowledge, a deficiency of knowableness. Science is founded upon facts, while nescience decreases as knowledge increases, the unknowable is diminished.

The principles of chiropractic science were not developed or evolved from any other method; they were discovered as pre-existing elements and formulated into a system. The principles which compose the science of chiropractic are as old as the vertebrata.

To know chiropractic as a science, we must become familiar with its principles, we must make it scientific. To know it as an art is to make it specific, make use of the knowledge which composes the science.

A chiropractor is one who has a knowledge of the science and art of chiropractic, one who is capable of performing the art of adjusting vertebrae; he should, also, comprehend the philosophy of the science and art, the reasons for so doing.

Science is the know-how; the art is the doing; the philosophy consists in the reasons why of phenomena, as explained by a knowledge of the powers and laws which govern them.

The science of chiropractic embraces the principles and demonstrated facts of biology.

The science of dynamics includes the principles and facts of machinery.

The science of chiropractic and that of machinery have no resemblance whatever, in their motive force. That being a fact, why try to illustrate either one by the principles belonging to the other? Just as well try to explain the science of grammar by that of astronomy; geography by mathematics; chemistry by agriculture; or that of music by navigation. Man is not a machine.

The science of chiropractic is in no way related to the science of machinery. Its phenomena are dependent upon vital force, not that of dynamics.

The structure of the body is defined under that of anatomy, not metalography—a treatise on metals.

Bodily functions depend upon vital force, not dynamics. The existence of metals, whether in the form of machinery or that of ore, depends upon certain inanimate qualities, whereas the existence of animals depends upon functions.

Vital philosophy and mechanical philosophy are not correlated, they are radically and entirely different.

The laws which govern the existence of animated beings and that of animated objects differ.

Chiropractic science is being enlarged and urged on to a higher development by the demands of the art of vertebral adjusting. Why not make use of the knowledge which composes the science?

In chiropractic, you should discriminate between science and art. Science depends upon principles, and art upon practice.

The theories of chiropractic become demonstrated facts, the practice an art.

Biology and chiropractic include vital phenomena in contradistinction to physical facts; those functions, energies and acts that depend upon life, as manifested by contrast to those which exist without intelligence.

A prominent writer aims to make a record in chiropractic by affirming that he is the author, formulator and constructor of the science of chiropractic; that the essence (the essential principles) is love, patience, perseverance, truth and equality; that these principles constitute its highest standard, wonderful beauty and simplicity. Love, patience, perseverance, truth and equality as principles belong to the Sunday School or the lodge room of some benevolent organization; as five principles they are not found among the 500 which the founder of chiropractic uses to compose its science.

Why not learn chiropractic as a science? Why not be specific in adjusting? Why not learn the specific cause of typhoid fever, acquire the knowledge of why, how and where adjust for it? Why not comprehend the how and the why organs and parts of the body are affected by displaced vertebrae? Why not know that hemiplegia is because of the displacement of the sixth dorsal vertebra, that one-half of the body may be affected by the fibers of that nerve? Why not become acquainted with the proper method of adjusting that vertebra? Why not learn of the two ganglionic chains of the sympathetic nervous system which reach from the occiput to the coccyx, its plexus of nerves extending into the cranium, the fibers of which unite with the cranial nerves, and that these vertebral cords are distributing agencies of organic life, reaching to all the viscera?

Why not learn that the neuro~~skeleton~~ is a protector of the central nervous system, and that when any portion thereof is displaced it is a disturber of vibration, heat and other functions? Why not learn to use the vertebral processes as levers to replace luxated vertebrae?

Science is knowledge, ascertained facts, accumulated, systematized information regarding causes and principles. Why not correlate and reduce to a system these principles; why not make them practical? Why not learn to reason from cause to effect? Why not become acquainted with physiological and pathological processes in health and disease?

Why not obtain knowledge regarding pyorrhea alveolaris; why not ascertain the fact that a discharge of pus from the margin of the gums, granulated eyelids, bleareyes, kidney affections, diseases of the sebaceous glands, and some headaches are because of a K. P. luxation, that two or more of these diseases may be associated, may result from over-tension on the fibers of one nerve which ramify the portions affected?

Why not be able to make a distinction between the diseased conditions arising from the tight, rigid, strained nerves of the third cervical and twelfth dorsal?

Why remain satisfied with a meager knowledge of the science, art and philosophy of chiropractic? Why not advance onward and upward toward perfection, why remain on the lower rounds, why not exert yourself and become eminent in your line of work instead of kicking down the ladder upon which others are climbing?

Nerve Vibration

The following is an answer to a 17-page article in the California Eclectic Journal, by Dr. E. P. Bailey of Los Angeles, Cal.

He says in part, "Lucky, indeed, shall we be if ever we succeed in throwing a gleam of light upon the modus operandi with which sense-impressions are communicated to the intellect, and transformed into thought or consciousness. The marvel does not exist in our having eyes and ears, but in our being able to see and hear. Explain this and perhaps you explain everything else that has hitherto puzzled our benighted understanding.

"And yet the whole mystery may admit of an explanation so simple that, when discovered, it will occasion universal surprise why nobody thought of it before."

NERVE VIBRATION.

Nerve vibration is associated with consciousness. Without it there would be no sensational intelligence, no activity which we recognize as life.

The phenomena of sound is produced by vibrations of the atmosphere. The vibrations impinge against the tympanum and continue inward over the acoustic, or auditory nerve. The tension of the tympanic membrane is not fixed as are stationary membranes; it is as well adapted for the reception of one vibration as another. In the absence of vibration a condition of relaxation exists. Our knowledge of unlimited variations of sound is recognized by the infinite diversity of nerve vibrations. Consciousness is determined by and must accord with acoustic vibrations.

Thought transference by speech is accomplished by and through the medium of atmospheric vibration. We recognize the volume and quantity of vibration focussed by the external ear and conducted to the acoustic nerve. The principles involved in the telephone and the ear are very similar; the phenomena of each are controlled by the same law. We recognize individual voices because of the difference in the vibratory movements. This is true whether conducted by the telephone wire or the atmosphere. We recognize the faces of individuals because of their dissimilarity, thus it is with voices. Faces and voices may be so distorted as to be unrecognizable. The combining of many voices, or that of many musical instruments, are blended into one vibration. Each instrument, or any combination of instruments, are presented and recognized by its peculiar vibration. The molecules of the atmosphere and those of the wire of the telephone transmit the vibratory movement. The diaphragm and the wire of the telephone perform the same office as

17

does the tympanum and the auditory nerve of the ear. The vibrations of the transmitting diaphragm are carried over the connecting wire, while those of the ear are vibrated over the cochlear and vestibular nerves, the two which form the auditory nerve, the eighth cranial. Nerve vibrations create consciousness. The vibrations of the atmosphere are impinged against the tympanum of the ear, transferred to the auditory nerve, and we recognize those vibratory movements.

The disagreeable popping of gas engines may be rendered noiseless by a set of discs so arranged as to deflect the vibrations causing them to whirl similar to the water in an eddy. Echo, a repetition of a sound. The reiteration is the oscillating waves of the atmosphere reflected. The energy expended in the rebound is sooner or later lost.

A stick of timber fifty feet long, more or less, is struck at one end, the vibratory movement of the molecules are transmitted from the end struck to all portions, even to every atom.

The particles of a tuning fork vibrate when struck. Its vibration is determined by the force of the stroke. Not only the particles of the fork vibrate, but the prongs move in a wave-like motion. This double movement of the atoms may be likened to waves of water which consist of an enormous amount of molecules, the drops of which move freely with each other, a good illustration of molecular oscillation. The vibrations of the tuning fork are communicated to the atmosphere, impinge against the tympanum of the ear, the mucous membrane is well supplied with the tympanum plexus of the glossopharyngeal nerve; these vibrations continue over the auditory nerve, are recognized by consciousness. The tuning fork is used to tone instruments. to get the pitch. Pitch is the rate of vibration. The vibrations of the voice is made to harmonize with those of the tuning fork.

I have just said that there are two separate and distinctly different movements of the atoms or molecules of substances. The movement of one atom against another, or others, for it touches all those which surround it, creates heat. The movement of a great number of these body atoms create within us consciousness.

Gould's Dictionary says, ''Temperature, the degree of intensity of heat or molecular vibration.''

Heat is a form of energy, this energy is created by motion. It is manifested in the effects of fire, the sun's rays and friction. The molecules (the smallest known particles of matter which move about as a whole) of all matter vibrate, that is, move to and fro, in a similar manner as the pendulum of a clock, or the balance wheel of a watch which vibrates four times in a second. The various degrees of temperature of iron are due to the amount of movement of the molecules of which it is composed. The varying temperature between that of 70 degrees and zero are due to molecular change (vibration) of its atoms. Energy traveling in the form of radiation is sometimes called radiant heat. Radiation, however, is not heat, it is the kinetic energy of vibrations of ether. By an increase or decrease in the movement of its particles the color and temperature are modified. The color of iron may be changed from black to that of red. By still increasing the movement of its particles the red color may be changed to that of white, and, by a yet greater agitation of its atoms the color becomes blue. The greater the vibration, the more active the molecules, the greater the heat.

When a resonant bar of metal is struck, made to respond to a certain amount of vibration, waves rush through the substance which are unlike in character to those vibrations going on all the time among the molecules. The molecular vibration of nerve tissue and wave motion differ in that the former is the movement of particles and the latter is of the whole.

The particles of all matter are always in a state of vibration. If inanimate matter changes its temperature according to the amount of its atomic vibration, why not living tissue? That the amount of nerve-tension determines the quantity of heat is a demonstrated fact. Bodily temperature may increase after death and run as high as 106 or even to 108 degrees. The heat of the body, whether normal temperature, inflammation or fever is a function of nerves. Nerves heat the body.

An impulse travels over a nerve by waves known as vibration, similar as a pulse-wave, only more rapid. The speed of thought (an impulse traveling over a nerve) has been duly measured by the aid of apparatus in physiological laboratories. In man the normal rate of vibration is said to be 114 feet per second. Sensory impulses, which convey sensation inward vary from 168 to 675 feet per second, the average being 282 feet. The commands, known as impulses, are carried over the nerves by vibration.

Why does death result from high temperature? Because excessive vibrations create sufficient heat to liquify tissue, necrose the web-like structure, render it too soft for normal vibration. The tripod of life, the vital tripod, the brain, heart and lungs, cease to innervate the organism through the nervous system, and maintain the circulation and aeration of the blood. If 200 nerve vibrations are normal, over that is an excess, heat is augmented, bones, nerves, blood vessels and other tissue become softened, changd in color from white to that of reddish-yellow, the vascular system softened, causing hemorrhage from rupture and perforation.

Nerves, like all material substances, are composed of particles, atoms or molecules, which vibrate, oscillate. When nerves are in a normal condition, known as tone—normal tension, normal elasticity and normal renitency—impulses are transmitted by vibration in a normal manner with the usual force. The amount of impulsive force is determined by the rate of transmission, the rate of action upon the quantity of vibration, and the amount of movement upon tension. Motor and sensory impulses are transmitted over the nervous system by molecular vibration. The force of an impulse depends upon its momentum, the momentum upon the impetus received from nerve vibration during transmission. If the nervous system is normal in its tension, vibrations are normal and the degree of temperature is that of 98 to 99 degrees.

Consciousness is associated with nerve vibration; the external organs focus the vibratory movements, perform the function of receiving, directing and transmitting vibrations. The retina of the eye and the tympanum of the ear respond to the vibrations of the atmosphere. These vibrations pass into the interior by means of the nervous system. If this means of communication is normal in tension, its vibration and carrying capacity are also normal. The tension and rigidity of nerve tissue determines the amount of molecular oscillation.

Petoskey, Mich., Aug. 13.—Miss Helen Keller, the noted blind and deaf girl, has heard her first note of music. She caught the vibrations of a violin string through her teeth, held against the bridge of the instrument, and, although her eardrums are useless, Prof. Frans Kohler of Oberlin conservatory declared today that the harmonies had been communicated to her brain and she had caught the strain. ''Like the voices of singing angels,'' said Miss Keller to Miss Macey, her teacher.

Light is transmitted by the vibration of ether at the rate of 186,300 miles per second. Vibrations strike the retina of the eye and are carried inward over the optic nerve. The retina forwards the vibratory impulses to the nerve which communicates between the brain and the organ of vision. The X-ray is a good illustration of light penetrating solid substances by ether vibration, yet it is not a therapeutical agent.

Air and ether are vibratory transmitting mediums. Ether interpenetrates the atmosphere, as well as all material substances, liquid or solid. Etheric vibrations pass freely through opaque bodies as light penetrates transparent substances, with the same velocity as that of light.

Ether penetrates all substances. Spirit permeates and inhabits all living bodies. Ether and spirit are not subject to laws which govern ponderable substances.

Telepathy, mental communication between two persons at a distance from each other without the aid of spoken or written signs, is accomplished through and by the transmitting vibratory qualities of ether. Ether is a medium filling all space, even in that which is occupied by fluids and solids. Its functions, so far as known, are the transmitting of light, the production of all the phenomena ascribed to electric, vital and magnetic force. Ether will in the near future play an important part in the transmission of thought, not only between individuals of this world, but between astral beings and those of the physical. Who knows

.t the way is now being opened for the inhabitants of other planets to converse with those of our own by the aid of etheric waves? The transmission of thought from planet to planet would be only an increase in distance as has been done with wireless telegraphy.

Molecular vibration is a law of the universe, nothing is exempt from this activity. It is universal in its application. Progression is an established principle. Spiritual progress toward perfection is dependent upon physcal and spiritual growth.

The universe is composed of spirit and matter. All living material is animated by spirit. The process of physical and spiritual growth are so intimately blended that it is difficult to separate one from the other. Our bodies are animated by spirit through molecular vibration; without vital force there would be no action guided by intelligence.

Astral spirits composed of supersensitive substance, inhabiting supersensible spheres are far more refined than the material of this world, yet they are undergoing a process of advancement analogous to that of individuals on this earth.

A Brief Review

Biology is the science of life. Life is intelligent action, movements guided by intelligence. Life exists because of renitency and elasticity of tissue; these conditions not only permit, make it possible to receive, but actually create a response to an impulse. Impulses are thoughts in transmission over the nervous system. In telepathy thoughts are transmitted by the vibrations of ether; in spoken language they are transferred by the vibrations of the air.

The soul is intelligent life; it is the product from uniting intelligence and material, spirit and body; the result of a combination of the immaterial with the material. Vital makes possible organic functions, the power of motion and feeling.

The amount of tension depends upon the relative position of the osseous frame, the neuroskeleton, the skeleton of the vertebrates.

Health is a condition wherein all the functions are performed with a normal amount of force. Disease is an existence in which the action of an organ or organs are improperly performed. Death is a situation wherein action has ceased to be controlled by intelligence. The state of dissolution, or the act of a rolling stone, is not that of intelligence. Inflammation is a condition in which some local portion exhibits a higher temperature than any other, including the blood. Do not forget, in order to disturb functions, there must be in-ordinate nerve tension, also, a change in heat production. Fever is a state in which the whole body is above normal in temperature. Fever is diffused inflammation. Inflammation is associated with corns; the heat of which may be diffused, if so, the patient has fever.

The neuroskeleton, when in normal position, is a protector of the nervous system, but, a nerve disturber when not properly placed.

PRESSURE. There are three kinds of pressure, impingement, pinch and stricture; two forms of injury, contusion and concussion; each are lesional.

Pressure on any portion of the nervous system (the encephalon, spinal cord, the ganglionic chains, ganglia or nerves) increases or impairs its carrying capacity of impulses (motor or sensory), causing too much or not enough functionating: heat is one of those functions.

To impinge is to press on one side. Impinging and impinge are verbs, they denote action, something to be done, are always followed by on, upon or against. A nerve may be impinged on, upon or against. Impingement is a noun, denotes the act or condition of being impinged on, upon or against.

22

Pinching or squeezing is an act done by pressure on two sides, a material placed between two harder substances.

Spinal Adjustment displays two cuts on pages 146 and 147; the former is designed to "show the normal condition of the intervertebral discs."

In anatomy a disc is a circular organ or body which is plate-like. The epiphyseal plates of bone are situated on the upper and under surfaces of the body of the vertebra and the intervertebral fibrocartilage are known as discs, because they are like a plate, flat and round.

The cut on page 147 is "Showing compressed intervertebral discs and an impinged nerve from narrowing of the foramina."

The term foramina should be foramen, as nerve is referred to in the singular number.

To compress is to press or squeeze together, to reduce in volume by pressure, to make more compact.

The intervertebral cartilage is a connective tissue, nonvascular, contains no nerves. It is surrounded by a fibrovascular membrane, in which blood vessels and nerves are freely distributed, by which it receives nutrition. It contains a fibrous element, its base being of chrondin, a viscous, jelly-like substance which may be separated from the fibrous portion by boiling.

In the living subject it may be destroyed, necrosed, by excessive heat. Inflammation of the surrounding membrane liquifies, liberates the gelatin and very often destroys the fibrous portion. Its size is not and cannot be reduced by compression as shown in the cut.

A displaced vertebra, one whose articular surfaces are separated, enlarges the foramina, therefore, does not occlude the opening, does not pinch, compress or squeeze the outgoing nerves as they pass through the intervertebral foramina. The spinal nerves and their branches may be impinged upon or against, or stretched because of displaced vertebra, but not pinched.

"Impinged nerves from narrowing of the foramina."

The author here refers to nerves being pinched, not impinged.

Constriction is a condition of being narrowed by a binding force applied around a tubular orrifice. A morbid contraction of a passage way, any hollow tube of the body. Constriction and stricture mean one and the same.

Illustrate stricture on board, contracture of nerve tissue, inflammation because of increased combustion of oxygen.

Compression is to press together, to make more compact, to reduce in volume, to make narrower in one direction.

A concussion is a shaking, a jarring, an agitation, or a shock caused by a collision.

The real and direct cause of disease is more or less nerve tension than normal. Displaced bones because of their pressure against, or nonresistance of nerves, or that of stretching, cause an extra or a lessened amount of tension.

An abnormal performance of function of the body is denominated disease, the kind depends upon the tissue affected and the function disturbed.

The subtile and nicely discriminating transmission of physiological impulses, in health, whether of cells, the elementary structure of which organic substances are formed, individual organs, or the body as an organism, is directed by an intelligence known as spirit.

Sensory nerves are those nerve-fibers which carry sensory impulses from the exterior inward, to a nerve-center, resulting in sensation. Sensation is the recognizance of nerve vibration. Sensory nerve centers is where nerve vibration is identified. A sensory nerve is an afferent nerve, one which transfers peripheral impressions to the sensoria, sense-centers. Sensory ganglia are those masses of nervous substance which are thought to serve as a center of nervous influence. The most prominent of the sensory nerves are those of the olfactory, optic, auditory, gustatory, tactile and thermal. To these should be added that of cenesthesia, conscious existence, painful or pleasurable, depression or exaltation, the general sense of bodily, or self-existence, the subconscious sensation by the functioning of the internal organs. Sensory impressions are the effects of external agents or bodies upon the organs of sense. These external agents or bodies are always the same, impulses as originated are always perfect, if the nervous system is in a normal condition, the impressions, afferent impulses, can not be otherwise than normal.

We have the spiritual and physical impulses, those from the creator and the mind. All efferent impulses are motor. All motor impulses, whether of the spirit or the mind, are normal, providing the nerves of transmission are of normal tension.

All thoughts, orders, commands, directions of the mind, known as impulses, are normal if voluntary, the lines of communication are normal.

All thoughts, orders, commands, directions of the spirit, a segment of the Universal Intelligence, contains in miniature all intelligence and qualities of the All-Wise Spirit, just as one drop of the ocean contains all the qualities of the briny deep.

All spiritual impulses, those which cause intelligent organic action, life, are perfect when originated, as much so as their creator, as manifested in the new-born babe which has not been injured, whose impulses are carried over nerves of normal tension; but, if the tension-frame is displaced, luxated ever so little, nerves stretched, vibration modified, innervation increased or decreased, we have conditions known as disease.

The body when diseased manifests no new functions, develops no new forms of energy, adds no new space or accommodation.

While the larger share of diseases, abnormal functionating, are because of trauma, toxine and autosuggestion, there are minor causes such as inhalation of gas, smoke or flame, lack of food, water or air, decompression of the atmosphere in tunnels and caisons, an excess or a deficiency of heat, local exposure to the extremes of heat or cold which induces necroses, and exposure to X-rays may lead to caries.

INFLAMMATION

Inflammation is from a Greek word which means a flame, to burn as a flame, a condition of being inflamed.

The early idea of inflammation was that of an entity and the treatment that of exorcism, adjuration or conjuration of evil spirits, expelling or driving out or off an evil spirit by using a holy name.

Pathologists state, inflammation is an inflammable condition, which like a fire must be subdued by appropriate means, such as antiphlogistines, counterirritants, venesection, cupping, leeching and the use of mercury. That inflammation is a local attempt to repair an injury. That inflammation is a local reaction to irritation, it tends to counteract an injurious agent and repair its deleterious effect. That inflammation is conservative in tendency, benign in disposition, the result of a carefully adjusted protective mechanism. That inflammation is a purifyer, a body cleanser.

The condition known as inflammation is brought about by disturbed tissue which have been damaged. The fact is, as demonstrated by the art of chiropractic, borne out by the principles of the science and the reasoning of its philosophy, inflammation and disturbed functions are the result of nerves being injured.

Inflammation is a condition wherein the function of heat is performed in too great a degree, the result of morbid nerve tissue.

Inflammation is recognized by redness, swelling, heat, pain, impaired functions, over renitent tissue and a change in catabolism.

Inflammation may be seated in any organ or tissue of the body wherein there are nerves. The hair, nails and cartilage are void of blood vessels and nerves, therefore are not subject to inflammation, neuritis or arteritis.

The part inflamed has a temperature much higher than the rest of the body. Blood has the same temperature throughout the vascular system.

Inflammation modifies physiological processes.

Some of our grandfathers believed that animal heat was furnished by a set of nerves which were known as calorific—heat furnishing. When the surrounding temperature was above 99 degrees, there was another set which they named frigerific—cold producing.

I am often told that anatomy cannot be otherwise than correct. I do not object to the slight difference in the number, form and structure of normal tissue found in different subjects, reversed organs, but I do disapprove of the physiological and pathological deductions. Grey says on page 846 of his 1910 edition, "Inflammation of the spinal cord (myelitis) may follow any of the acute specific fevers." Fever is diffused inflamma-

26

tion. There can be no fever without a local inflammation. Inflammation always precedes fever. The sensible phenomena indicating inflammation are redness, heat, pain, swelling and disordered function. Redness because of excess of blood containing the red corpuscles; heat because of nerve excitation, contraction and excessive vibration; pain is a sensation confined to nerves only; inflamed nerves are swollen, enlarged in their diameter and contracted lengthwise; functions are disordered because of disturbed nervous tissue, normal function depends upon normal amount of energy, an impulse given too much force or a lack of arouses too much latent energy or not enough.

We are told by pathologists that the pain and swelling are because of congestion. Pathologists look to blood as a functional disturber. If a disturber it should also be a corrector. The blood is one of the four liquids of the body, the only one which circulates; the other fluids osmose, transudate through moist membranes.

Dunglison says, ''Inflammation is not easily defined.'' If pathologists knew that heat was a function of nerves, the cause and the condition of inflammation would be easily accounted for and explained. Such knowledge would let in a flood of light on the etiology of many diseases now given as obscure.

Blood circulates; serum, lymph and chyle, osmose, transudate, pass through a moist membrane.

Artero-sclerosis in old age is physiological. In youth and adult life it is pathological.

Post mortem examinations show but little of which we desire to know. Examine the living subject for benefit and information.

Neuritis, nerve inflamed, sensitive to the touch, hardened, enlarged diametrically and contracted lengthwise. Microscopic examination shows myelin sheaths, swollen fibers (filaments, axis cylinders). Owing to the number of fibers we may have multiple neuritis. Filaments of one nerve may leave it and join another. Neuritis changes the structure of nerves. Arteritis modifies the structure of arteries.

Inflammation is present in most, if not all diseases, in the acute if not the chronic.

Inflammation of the mucous membrane causes catarrh of any canal, cavity or hollow organ which communicates externally by an aperture through the skin.

Nerve contraction causes an undue amount of heat, gall stones, hardened ear wax and dropsy are because of inflammation.

The healing of wounds and fractures require a rise in temperature in order to furnish a larger per cent. than usual of the red corpuscles.

The degree of general temperature determines the per cent of red and white corpuscles. Local temperature determines the per cent of red or white and the amount of leakage deposited.

Necrotic inflammation causes death of tissue; softened tissue has little or no vibration, the carrying quality of impulses.

Inflammation is characterized by excessive emigration of leukocytes from the blood vessels, which soon disappear by colliquative necrosis.

Arteritis is an inflammation of an artery, the nervi vasorum is irritated, inflamed. Blood vessels rupture because of being softened. Softening and hardening are known as malacia and sclerosis.

Many persons suffer in an amputated limb, because the pressure, the cause of pain and other diseased conditions, has not been removed.

"Blood poisoning, septicemia, pyemia, toxemia," are medical terms used to account for any ailment which is presumed to arise from introduction of decomposed organic matter into the blood, excrementitious toxins of the intestinal canal not properly eliminated, putrefactive microorganic germs which grow and multiply in the blood.

In the above pathological conditions, please remember, morbid tissue and abnormal functionating always accompany each other. It is impossible for either to exist without the other. "Blood poisoning" will be found coexisting with a more or less intense nervous irritation known as inflammation, a tissue necrosis. The tissue shows very marked alterations, the cells or intercellular substance is softened and disintegrated.

While it is a fact that inflammation causes abnormal organic manifestation, there are no new functions developed. Physiological acts have become pathological.

We are now back to the elementary proposition, nerves heat the blood, as well as all parts of the body. Hyperthermia changes the amount of and the per cent. of the solid substances of the blood, the corpuscles. Behind all abnormal functions, is the change in the structure of nerve tissue and an increase or decrease of nerve vibration.

The following quotations were clipped from The Los Angeles Times of August 17, 1912.

"Cold feet and cold hands—other things being equal these indicate poor circulation."

I presume that circulation refers to the blood, as no other fluid of the body circulates, makes a circuit. The blood remains the same temperature throughout the body regardless of the feet and hands being cold or warm. The blood is the same temperature in the warm hands and the cold feet; the same blood circulates throughout the body about seventy times a minute.

"You should eat nourishing food and make good blood and enough of the starches, sweets, and fat to make heat."

If it takes nourishing food to make good blood, then bad blood would be the result of eating unnutritious food. "What is one man's food is another man's poison."

Dr. Warman follows the above with morning and evening exercises the hands and feet. Exercise excites the nervous system, causing an increase of vibration, consequently increased heat.

A. T. Still, the founder of osteopathy, says, on page 74 of his work, that bad blood is the cause of fibroid tumors, painful monthlies, constipation, diabetes and dyspepsia. The founder of chiropractic states that, nerve impingement, pressure against nerves, and more or less nerve tension than normal, is the cause of these diseases—quite a difference between osteopathy and chiropractic. Food furnishes material for the production of living tissue; it embraces those substances which are necessary for the maintenance and composition of the body. Bad blood is defined by pathologists as a deficiency in quanity, or a lack of the proper amount of red corpuscles. Pernicious anemia, a deficient amount of blood, or a deficiency in the relative number of red corpuscles, is a pathological condition which does not depend upon the amount of, or the quality of the food taken, but upon the temperature of the body. It is true, ingesta which irritates, acts as a poison on the nervous system, modifies the activity of molecular oscillation and increases heat production. The circulation of the blood and its quality depend upon the condition of the nervous system.

Medical practitioners state, an anemia may be due to an insufficient amount of food, excessive drain, exhausting discharges, blood-waste, hemorrhages, action of poisons, idiopathic (no known or recognized cause), and the cause is often obscure.

Traumatic injuries and poisons affect nerve plexuses which are freely distributed on the surface and into the substance of the heart, the nervi vasorum surrounding the arteries and veins, supplying the media (middle coat) with a network of nerve fibers which form dense plexuses giving them the power of contractility. This function of shortening into a more compact form, a power possessed by living muscle-fibers and the nervous tissue, is modified by poisons and the displacement of the neuroskeleton.

VERTEBRAL LUXUATIONS

In pathology luxation and dislocation mean one and the same.

A luxation is a displacement (not misplacement) of two or more bones whose articular surfaces have lost, wholly or in part, their natural connection.

Pathologists give two causes for luxations, one known and the other unknown. The known is caused by accidental luxations, owe their existence to external violence; the unknown to spontaneous luxation, those which owe their displacement to diseased conditions of the joint, including the vertebrae, known as tuberculosis; the bones and joints are affected with strumous arthritis, indolent ulcers, or that of white swelling, gelatinous arthritis, attended with slight continued fever; the cause of the morbidity is obscure, therefore said to occur of itself without any manifest external cause.

Diseases are said to be spontaneous which have no apparent cause, occurring without any external influence. For example, intra-uterine amputation, congenital dislocation and fracture. As fast as the causes become known they are taken out of the list of spontaneous abnormalities. Chiropractic has greatly lessened this list.

Luxations are complete when the bones have entirely lost their natural connection; incomplete when they partly retain it; and compound when a wound communicates with the displaced joint.

Chiropractors are concerned with the incomplete luxations, articular surfaces slightly displaced and the relative position they occupy toward each other.

The vertebral column has four normal curvatures. The cervical and lumbar bend anterior, while the dorsal and sacral have their curvatures posterior. A lordosis is an angular curvature of the cervical or lumbar portion of the spine. A kyphosis is an angular curvature of the dorsal portion of the spine, the sacral curvature being fixed and permanent owing to the vertebrae being fused. Scoliosis is a lateral curvature. An abnormal curvature consists of a sudden angular break, an increase in the convexity of the normal bend, a separation of the articular surfaces of two adjoining vertebrae, the superior articular processes of one or both sides being driven or drawn backward and away from its mate. Displacements cause a stretched condition of the spinal nerves, or some one or more of their branches, or the sympathetic, ganglinated, vertebral cords. A displacement of the twelfth dorsal (the spinous process of which is displaced anterior of the axial line of the vertebral column) not only affects certain organs and portions of the body, because of excessive tension created, but, also, a portion or all of the spinal column through

30

excessive heat, softening the vertebrae, causing anterior, posterior and lateral curvature, owing to the portion of the vertebral bodies softened and narrowed. As displacement of the twelfth dorsal caused abnormal curvature, replacing it in its normal position will restore the vertebral column to its normal curve. I have, in twenty-six years, only met one exception to the above mentioned abnormal curvatures, that of Miss Pearl Weeks, which was returned to normal by adjusting the twelfth dorsal, the rule holding good even in reversed scoliosis and lordosis. Any angular curvature, displacement of a spinous process posteriorly by the racking of a vertebra from its normal alignment, can be replayed by hand, using the spinous process as a lever.

There are three forms of abnormal spinal curvatures, each of which has a different cause. The angular curvature consists of a break, a separation of the articular processes between two vertebrae. A curvature known as Pott's disease, carries of the spine, supposed by pathologists to be of tuberculous origin. The curvature which has no knuckle, no sharp break nor vertebral caries, but, an increased curvature in the cervical, dorsal or lumbar, or in both of the latter two, from the vertebrae becoming wedge-shaped.

Displaced vertebrae, by impinging or stretching, cause contraction of nerve tissue. Tension is the condition of being stretched. Tension, more or less than normal, causes an increase or decrease of vibration, which means a greater or less force of an impulse and a corresponding amount of heat.

Nerve contraction increases vibration, irritation and heat. The force of an impulse is augmented by the greater speed in transit. The bounding back of an impulse is known as reflex action. The greater the renitency (the bounding back), the greater is energy aroused as expressed in the performance of function.

Displaced bones cause pressure upon nerves and consequent tension and deranged function. Slight deflections of vertebrae cause pressure on the nerves given off by the spinal cord, functional derangements are the result. By restoring them to their normal position, normal function is restored.

Nerve fibers possess the property of conducting impulses outward and inward. The amount of impulsive force is determined by the rate of transmission, the rate of that action upon the quantity of vibration and the amount of that movement upon tension. Physiological and pathological activity between peripheral end-organs and their central connection is dependent upon nerve tension. The specific energy of a nerve is due to its anatomical structure, its elasticity and tension.

A nerve pressed upon by a fractured or a luxated bone would be stretched were it not for the responsive principle of life which resists pressure. The impulsive force normally conveyed by the nerve is modified by the elastic resistance known as renitency. The result is either too much or not enough function, conditions known as disease. The contraction and expansion of the nervous system has a normal limit known as tone, the basis upon which I founded the science of chiropractic. Any deviation therefrom is recognized as disease. Tone denotes normal temperature, normal structure, normal tension and normal vibration of nerves.

An angleworm, when relaxed, may measure six inches. Press against it, impinge upon it, try to stretch it and immediately a response of increased tension is observed; it contracts lengthwise and its diameter is increased. This ability of elastic resistance to any opposing force is an inherent quality of all living matter. Dead material does not possess it. An impingement upon a nerve calls into action two opposing forces. The impigning body tends to stretch the nerves, while the inherent principle of self-preservation exerts an activity toward contracting it.

Trauma the cause of disease, increasing or decreasing function, is direct in displacing osseous tissue. Poisons as causes are indirect, they act on nerves, nerves on muscles, their combined action draw vertebrae out of alignment.

Autosuggestion may be therapeutical, curative, or morbific, causing hysteric paralysis, contraction of muscles, impairment of vision, convulsions, sensory disturbances and psychic manifestations. A change of thought is restful, but a constant continuation of the same thought, using the selfsame nerves, causes nerve disturbance and some form of insanity, and yet there is no discernable lesion of the nervous system.

The relationship existing between bones and nerves are so nicely adjusted that any one of the 200 bones, more especially those of the vertebral column, cannot be displaced ever so little without impinging upon or stretching adjacent nerves. Pressure upon nerves, agitates, creates an excess of molecular vibration, the effects of which when local, are known as inflammation, when diffused as fever. Nerves are the conveyors of impulses which create functions; an increase of vibration causes an excess of function—local inflammation or fever—symptoms which are common to most diseases.

Subluxated vertebrae disarrange the costo-central articulation, the juncture of the head of the rib with the vertebra. These projecting surfaces press against and impinge upon one or more of the four branches of the spinal nerve.

The Adjuster contains thirty-six pages, from 189 to 225, devoted to luxations, giving the opinions of many authors. Please read them carefully and notice how near they came to getting onto chiropractic in its principles, art and philosophy.

Health, Disease, Life and Death.

What do scientists, philosophers and divines know of life and death? What knowledge have you of the relation existing between intelligence and material, spirit and matter? Is not death an incident of life?

What is life, disease, death and eternal intelligent existence? What force created this human organism? What is this intelligent vital agency and from whence does it come? What of this intellectual entity which continues our existence as an intelligent living being? These questions have been propounded by savants of all ages. Chiropractors are able at least in a great measure, to answer these very important questions.

My ideas concerning health, disease, life and death have been greatly modified by years of careful research.

Health is that condition of the body in which all the functions are performed in the usual manner, impulses forwarded over the nervous system at the usual rate, giving the proper force to the rebound (reflex action) of the renitent tissue, all acts being performed in a normal degree.

The nervous system is the line of communication of our thoughts (impulses). Impulses are not fluids which flow. When the nervous tissue is normal in its structure, tension, firmness and renitency have the degree of tone, the transference of thought, commands (impulses) are of normal force, the result of health.

Disease has always been considered and treated as an entity, a being with an intelligence, one which could be talked to, commanded to go at our bidding. The body treated in such a manner with drugs and incantations, so as, to make it uncomfortable for its habitation. Disease is a condition.

We are learning to think aright. Instead of a fearful reverence for irrational superstition, we are learning to reason along biological lines.

In order to give you an idea of advancement in correct reasoning, the difference between superstition and rationalism, I will quote one illustration of the former from each of four old books I have.

Bate's Dispensatory by William Salmon, Professor of Physic, date 1694, containing "His choice and select recipes, applicable to the whole practice of physic and chyurgery, with above five hundred chymical processes, those so much famed in the world." On page 897 he gave the formula for "The Sympathetic Ointment" for wounds. The prescription is preceded by the ℞ which was then, as well as now, always placed at the commencement of a recipe. Dunglison's Dictionary says of this ℞ "Originally it was the sign of Jupiter, and was placed at the top of a

33

formula to propitiate the king of the gods, that the compound might act favorably.''

Jupiter was the ancient Italian god of the heavens.

The compound was made of ''Oil of roses, linseed oil, man's grease, moss of a man's skull, killed by a violent death in powder, mummy, man's blood, mix and make an ointment. By this ointment all wounds are healed; anointing the instrument by which the wound was made, once a day, every day, if the wound be great, otherwise, if the wound be small, once every second or third day may suffice. The weapon is to be kept wrapt up in a clean linen cloth, and in a place not too hot, lest the patient suffers thereby.''

Physicians of the past and present in selecting portions of humans or animals always take those of the male as they are supposed to make stronger drugs than those of the females. They chose those who had met violent death, for the reason that those dying of disease would sow the germs of destruction. They treated the instrument as the producer and repairer.

The London Dispensatory, date 1716, on page 169, gives a valuable (?) recipe.

''The hair of the patient made into a powder and drank cures the jaundice. The ashes of it mixt with hog's lard as an ointment helps luxated joints; the simple ashes stop bleeding. An oil distilled from it with honey, anointed on bald places, causes hair to grow.

''The finger nails of the patient made into a powder or infusion cause vomiting, great sickness at the stomach, and giddiness in the head; the powder laid to the navel in dropsies, is said to cure them.

''To cure consumption, take the hair and nails of the patient, cut them small, and put them in a hole in the root of a cherry tree, and then stop it with clay. To cure quartans (fever) and the gout, take the said hair and nails, cut small, and either give them to birds in a roasted egg, or put them into a hole bored into the body of an oak tree, or else mix them with wax, and stitch it to a live crab, casting it into the river again.''

The above while relieving (?) the patient of the evil was hard on the trees, crabs and birds.

The people of Europe and America are making foolish pother over Friedman's serum evolved from a turtle as a cure of tuberculosis. I recall to memory Brown-Sequard's elixir of life, Dr. Kochs consumption serum. Koch had found the wiggler and the dope that would stop his wiggling.

The above are but the survival of the old superstition, ''The hair of the dog that bit you will heal the wound.''

In 1776 Baron van Swieten, counsellor and first physician to their majesties the Emperror and Empress of Germany; perpetual president of the College of Physicians in Vienna; member of the Royal Academy of Sciences and Surgery at Paris; H. Fellow of the Royal College of Physicians at Edinburgh, published a book. On page 37 he says, "A pleurisy terminates either in a cure, in other diseases, or in death. This is a circumstance which a pleurisy has in common with all other diseases." The Baron had made a wonderful discovery, that persons affected with disease either got well or died, unless their affections ended in some other disease.

Samuel Frederick Gray published a treatise on pharmacology in 1824. On page 159 he says, "In a medical or chemical point of view, animals are inferior in rank to vegetables, as neither affording remedies of such power, nor consisting of so many distinct principles, as the latter.

"There is even reason to suppose that most of the virtues attributed to animal substances are imaginary, and that their apparent effects ought to be ascribed to the other substances exhibited in them. In general, we only mention those substances, which are, or rather have been, kept in the shops.

"Human skull. Cranium hominis. The powder is used in epilepsy: those which have been long buried are to be preferred; and some even limit the effect to that triangular bone called the os triquetrum (os triangulare, cuneiform bone of the wrist)." Age and distance lend enchantment to superstition.

Hundreds of scientists are devoting their lives to the study of bacteriology, germ investigation, a microscopical branch of biology, in order to determine their relation to health and disease, not realizing that life action is due to the combination of intelligence and matter, spirit manifestation through material.

The isopathic theory and system of treatment of disease by means of the causal agent, that it is possible to cure a disease by means of the virus of the same disease; also, the treatment of a diseased organ, that its abnormal functions may be returned to normal by an extract of the same organ from a healthy animal, the curing a diseased organ by eating the analogous organ of a healthy animal, savors of canibalistic barbarism, eating an enemy transfers his fighting qualities to the devourer. "The explanation of this natural immunity is still uncertain." "All the phenomena of immunity have not been satisfactorily explained." Medical men, who believe in this dogma, think natural immunity hereditary, that thon's ancestors were immunized as a result of being infected. The immunity being transmitted to their descendants. "But little is known regarding the antitoxins." The theory is, the serum of one animal when introduced into the blood of another may destroy or modify the form, nature and structure of the red corpuscles." "This wonderful protective adaptation of the body toward the invasion of foreign cells; the nature of the processes involved is not at all understood, the phenomena is, therefore, designated provisionally as a biological reaction."

By referring to Dunglison's Medical Dictionary, date 1903, page 1100, you will find that animal extracts are yet in vogue.

Disease consists of a change in structure, position or function. Disease is a disturbed condition, functions performed abnormally, in too great a degree or not enough; it is not something foreign to the body which by some means enters it; it is not a thing of enmity which we have to fight.

Disease does not involve any new functional expression which it did not already possess. Disease is a manifestation of too much or not enough energy. Energy is liberated force; in the living being it is known as vital force.

A normal amount of energy released from that which is stored, results in health. The amount of energy stored for future use depends upon the condition of the organ as a storage receptacle. Disease is the result of releasing too much or not enough stored energy. Energy is the latent power or force in an organ, which when released creates action. Energy is aroused by a motor impulse; if the impulse is normal in force then the normal amount of energy is expended. Disease is abnormal functionating—not enough or too much action—too much or not enough life. Life consists of intelligent action. Disease is morbid tissue and abnormal functionating. The quality of tissue and the amount of functionating are coexistent. In all diseases we find an excess of, or a diminished amount of energy (force) expended.

In one lesson I cannot fully cover the cause of disease, as it takes in a large amount of chiropractic education in principles and facts regarding the science of biology.

Abnormal structure cannot do otherwise than be the creator of disease.

Death is natural, whether of a physiological or a pathological nature —it is a natural result, a natural change, all laws are of nature, natural.

What is that which is present in the living body and absent in the dead? It is an intelligent force, which I saw fit to name Innate, usually known as spirit. It creates and continues life when the vital organs are in a condition to be acted upon by that intelligence.

RACHITIS OR RICKETS

Rachitis, plural rachises, is a Greek word meaning spine.

The origin of the word rickets is uncertain. It means to twist, to sprain.

Rachitis and rickets are synonymous terms, meaning one and the same.

Rachitis is an inflammatory disease of the vertebral column. This is an interesting and instructive condition for chiropractors to study.

Medical dictionaries, pathological and orthopedic works describe definitely the malformation of the bones, degeneration of the organs, general feverishness and abnormal functionating.

Rachitis or rickets is a disease of early childhood characterized by defective nutrition of the entire body and alterations in the growing bones. The prominent symptoms are restlessness, fever, profuse sweating, and general sensitiveness, associated with characteristic skeletal lesions. The head becomes bulky, the spinal column curved, the sternum projected, and the long bones bent.

Physicians and surgeons are not decided as to the cause or causes. They have many and varied speculative opinions.

When it becomes generally known that heat is a function of nerves, chiropractic beams of enlightment will revolutionize the practice of medicine and make visible that which is now obscure. A natural insight of your teacher, untrammeled by superstition or education, assisted by revelation and an investigation from a chiropractic viewpoint has enabled him to throw an illuminating light on the etiology of this heretofore mysterious disease.

In the Adjuster, on pages 237 to 255, is given a full description by many authors of this ''constitutional and nutritive disorder.''

It is my desire to make you and the world acquainted with the etiology of this well-known disease, characterized by disorders of the digestive system and alterations in the shape and structure of bones.

Osteomalacia and rickets are similar in some respects and yet quite dissimilar in others.

Rachitis is a disease of childhood, osteomalacia (softening of bones) is of adult life. The former is present while bones are being constructed, while the latter is only found after bones are formed.

The structure of all tissue, more especially that of nerves, is modified as age advances. The same pressure upon, or tension of the same nerves at different ages produce quite different effects, which are classed as different diseases. No two of us look alike, no two have nerves of the same quality in health, while in disease these differences are augmented.

The primary and secondary qualities of the nervous system differ in individuals regarding their size, figure, number, situation, molecular action, and more especially in intellecutal perception, the quality and character of which is formed by contact with the five senses of consciousness.

The structure and composition of bones undergo a change as age advances. Those of a child are composed of three parts gelatine and one part phosphate of lime, bone matter; in old age the proportion is reversed, one part gelatine to three parts of bone material. Herein is the reason why the bones of the aged do not knit so readily when fractured as in those of younger years.

Hyperthermia, excessive heat, temperature above normal, creates a larger per cent. of the red corpuscles and a corresponding inadequate number of the white corpuscles. This increase of the erythrocytes and the lessening of leukocytes has a tendency to soften all tissue, more noticeably bones and nerves.

The solid portion of the body is about one-tenth of the whole. The normal per cent of the red and white corpuscles are variously given as 300 to 600 of the red to one of the white. The color of the blood is from the preponderance of the red corpuscles. The corpuscles are the solid portion of the blood and constitute about one-third to one-half of the blood. In anemia the number of the red may be reduced to one-tenth of the usual number. In fever there is an increase of the colored and a lessening of the colorless corpuscles; during convalescence this order is reversed. In the healing of wounds and fractures the temperature of the body is physiologically increased in order to produce plastic material, which is cartilage-like, known as callus, the osseous substance deposited in and around the divided portions of a fractured bone. A portion of this callus becomes perminent and is changed into true bone, the temporary or provisional callus, is used as a splint to keep the ends of the bones in apposition; when the union is complete it is removed by absorption. Poisons change the relative per cent of the red and white corpuscles, whether more or less depends upon the increase or decrease of organic function. Poisons affect nerves, cause a greater or lessened tension, raise or lower the temperature, modify the per cent of red and white corpuscles. The pus cells of an abscess consist of dead white corpuscles. Excess of heat makes it unfavorable for their existence and favorable for the red.

Scurvy and rachitis may be associated. A pathologist says, "We know nothing concerning the pathogenesis of scurvy."

In all diseases wherein a high temperature was maintained before death, the bones and marrow will be found of a reddish color, owing to an excess of the red corpuscles and a corresponding deficiency of the white. If the temperature falls below normal, remaining so for a time, there will be an excess of the leukocytes and a lessening of the erythrocytes.

A very high temperature causes an increase in the vascular circulation and an increased tension of the nervi vasorum (nerves distributed to the walls of blood vessels) in the perivascular (around) tissue.

Varying degrees of temperature represent a corresponding rate of molecular oscillation, a greater or less vibration of atoms.

Substances known as poison are noxious because of their exciting or depressing effects on the nervous system and their adaptation to modify functions; for this reason and for such a purpose physicians prescribe drugs.

Any ingesta which causes abnormal functionating is a poison. The continued use of one article of food may act as a poison upon the nervous system in a like manner (a lack of rest, a continued strain) as does autosuggestion in hysteria, insanity and neurasthenic affections. Autosuggestion may relax nerves, or act as a tensor.

The heat condition of caries and rachitis are different in that the former is local, while the latter is diffused. In necrosis and caries the heat is circumscribed, in the latter it is dispersed.

Why not learn to make the distinction between the diseased conditions arising from the tight, rigid, strained nerves of the third cervical and those of the twelfth dorsal?

In bone softening without disintegration, the general diffusion of heat is due to hypertension of the twelfth pair of dorsal nerves, the second center place. In necrosis and caries the heat is localized because of tension on other nerves than those of the twelfth dorsal, which may be determined by the area affected. Caries, necrosis, rachitis and osteomalacia are due to the function of heat being performed in excess, because of the displacement of some portion of the neuroskeleton.

All rachitic conditions are because of displacement of the twelfth dorsal vertebra; this is an established fact: then, why not replace it, thereby restoring those nerves to normal tension; tension depending upon the position of the bones of the neuroskeleton. It takes time to create abnormal curvatures, misshapen vertebrae—it will take time to reshapen them back to normal; this may be accomplished by proper daily adjusting.

Stover's case of ichthyosis congenita, dry scaly tetter, a skin disease, a squamous scale-like covering from the sebaceous glands, which disappeared in summer and re-appeared in winter, covered the posterior portions of the forearms and the dorsal region of the back, also, pyorrhea alveolaris, inflammation of the alveolar periosteum, looseness of the teeth, shrinkage and suppuration of the gums, cancer of the tongue and supposed consumption were relieved by adjusting the twelfth dorsal for the former two diseases and the fifth dorsal for the latter two conditions.

BIOLOGY

In all the affairs of life we prosecute careful investigation in order to determine exactly what are the facts. Thinking we are right does not of necessity constitute righteousness. Thinking right or wrong is a matter of education. The standard of truthfulness may be quite different from the view we may happen to have. If, for example, I had gotten the idea that two times three are seven and carry that erroneous multiplication into all of my arithmetical calculations, architectural and financial operations; the fact that such was my honest conception would not undo or make right the erroneousness of my figuring.

We should think correctly in order that we may get at facts. In chiropractic, too many teachers manufacture their own definition of terms, make a dictionary according to thon's conception. What would be the result if each banker and broker should invent and persist in using his own devised addition and multiplication table. Herein arises the discordant, inharmonious jangling among chiropractors regarding what constitutes the principles of the science, the method of adjusting, palpation and nerve tracing, the philosophy of the science and the art.

Biology presents only facts, the laws of which are of nature, natural, whether exhibited in health or disease. As chiropractors we should continue to advance toward the truth in order to bring ourselves into closer relation with eternal realities. A truthful statement of facts is correct, not because of our consideration, supposition or imagination, but because it IS right, because it conforms with everlasting truth.

All is nature, natural, there is nothing supernatural, phenomena may be superusual and supernormal. Any observable fact or event may appear miraculous when it is merely marvelous; it is because of our ignorance in regard to nature's law that they appear so to us.

Bio—a combining form from the Greek Bios, life, used to indicate relation to, or connection with, life, vital phenomena, or living organisms.

Biology is the science of life, the study of living beings. It consists of a knowledge of principles and facts concerning life—the certainty that we live and the conditions which cause us to have an intelligent existence. Life may be one of health or one of disease. Biology treats of organized beings under their diverse relations, their organic structure, life, growth, action and reproduction. I desire to give you some of the important principles of biology as observed from several view points, confining myself to the physiological branch which treats of the functions of the human body. You may accuse me of repetition. Fleeting impressions are only veneered. Essential ideas are worthy of repetition.

40

What is life? It is that quality which distinguishes a living animal or plant from an inorganic body, from one which does not live, whose movements are not determined by an intelligence. Life consists of actions guided by intelligence.

Life may consist of too much elastic force, too great or a lack of resisting vigor, such a condition is known as disease.

Animals and plants have an existence because they live; they exist as living beings on account of their bodies being composed of organs controlled by an intelligence. An organ is any part of an organism; an organism is an organized being. An organized being is one which is composed of organs. An organ is that which has a particular function to perform. The sensory or sense organs receive impressions from objective realiites through the sensory or sense organs, transform them into sensation—conscious sense perception. Eyes are organs of sight, ears that of hearing, the olfactory organ has the sense of smell, the nerves of taste are distributed to the palate, epiglottis, larynx and the tongue. To these may be added the senses of pressure, temperature, pain, hunger and thirst.

Biology in its broadest sense includes embryology, the development of the embryo in animals and plants; zoology, the form, nature and habits of animals; botany deals with plant life; physiology relates to the functions of living bodies, animals or plants; anatomy, the dissection of organized bodies, whether human, brute-animal, or vegetable; cytology, the science of cell life. In common language it includes the principles and facts of the origin, development, structure, functions and distribution of plants and animals. Life exists because of the exercise of organs. Physiologists study functions, the action of organs. Physiology deals with the processes, activities and the phenomena incidental to life, the characteristic actions which constitute life, those qualities which determine a living organism from one which does not live, those actions which depend upon an intelligence.

Life consists of the actions of a living organism, they may be of health, those desired to make us happy, give us ease, or they may be those known as disease, those which cause sensation and actions not desired.

The body is incapable of creating new forces. Force is that which originates or arrests motion. Vital force is the energy which gives life or action to an organism, the vital power which distinguishes living matter from the dead. Organic force is the inherent vigor latent in an organ. Nerve force is the power or ability to conduct impulses. Reserve force is the energy which is stored in an organ or organism that is not required for normal functionating. Intelligent actions are the expressions of the sum total of life. This intelligence is able to accumulate and store energy derived from without. Certain fixed and definite conditions release this energy.

The condition of an organ suitable for health is known as tone. Tone consists of normal tension, normal firmness and normal renitency. When nerves have the proper tension, the suitable solidity and the required resisting force, health is the result.

Biology embraces a knowledge of living matter in contradistinction to substances which do not possess that vital force directed by an intelligence, a quality essential to intelligent beings.

Physiology treats of the functions which create and continue a living existence, one which is normal, congenial and of health. Pathologic physiology is that condition in which the functions are performed abnormally.

Pathology treats of the modifications of functions and the changes of tissue coincident therewith which always accompany the disturbance of functions. Pathology includes functions performed in an unusual manner, also changes in position from that of normal, as well as, abnormal structure of organs.

The philosophy of chiropractic, the reasons concerning the science and art, is an explanation of the phenomena of life in health and disease.

The principles of biology are those of chiropractic; their associated elements constitute the science of chiropractic; when formulated they express in a clear and definite form the scientific part of chiropractic. Chiropractic science is identified by the principles of biology; its existence depends upon biological self-evident facts; they are the constituent elementary parts. To comprehend chiropractic it is essential that we should know of biology, the science of life, the physiological action of organs. We are, therefore, especially interested in that branch of knowledge which deals with the activities and phenomena incidental to and characteristic of living organisms. The science of chiropractic, the principles and facts pertaining to life, are distinct from anatomy, that branch of knowledge which deals with the structure only. In consideration of the above I would give much more time to the study of the science of chiropractic than to that of anatomy. The medical fraternity have studied tissue structure for centuries and yet did not become acquainted with the practical application of the principles which compose the science of chiropractic.

The power or faculty of receiving impressions through the five senses is from without, is of the animal functions, not organic.

While in the new-born organic life is perfect, physical life is not yet manifested. The faculty of receiving mental impressions through the action of sense organs is one of education. Actions known as organic are not of education.

The vital organs perform each their normal function from the first; the animal functions have to be developed. The recently born child has eyes to see, but it sees not; ears to hear, but it hears not; hands to grasp, but they do not grip; legs to walk, but they do not take a step. It has a mouth to suck by which it imbibes nutrition. The taking of sustenance is imperative for the continuance of life, therefore it may be considered an organis function directed by the creator, the intelligence which directs, controls and builds the body. The entire organism is devoted to sustaining life. To discern what is food and what is not, the senses of taste and smell are present at birth, even so in the child born a month or two before the proper time. The child shows satisfaction or disgust with ingesta which is pleasant or unpleasant to the taste, as shown by its facial expression, which is not acquired or imitative. As the infant advances in age its face becomes more expressive, its liking for sweet food continues during lactation, also a dislike for that which is sour.

To be a food in a physiological sense the substance must not affect injuriously the nutritive process by which food stuff is transposed into tissue. In the infant sugar is needed to form fat, furnish elasticity to muscles and nerves. In diabetes the sugar is carried out of the system, in consequence of which the patient becomes quite thin and emaciated. Carbohydrate fat is of a more solid consistency than the fat derived from other sources. The physiological assimilation of sugar in the production of fat is a vital organic process and cannot be imitated in the laboratory. The human milk contains a ratio of one of albumen, two of fat and 4.2 of sugar. Acids as ingesta produce rigor, rigidity, shortening of nerves and muscles. Emotional states of the mother modify the quantity and quality of milk, indicating the connection between the mammary glands and the nervous system. Innate, the spirit, selects that which contains sugar instead of acids. To the infant acids create a toxic effect, a pathological condition, contraction of the nervous system. It will be readily seen why the controlling intelligence selects substances which are sweet instead of sour.

The sense of smell is closely allied to that of taste. The nose often suggests to the mouth whether to accept or reject an article for ingesta.

Feeling is first experienced and manifested through the lips. What the adult would feel with the hands, the infant tries with its lips and mouth. Feeling with the lips is followed by sensing with the hands and feet, stuffing everything reachable into its mouth to feel and taste. In time sight and hearing are developed. While sight gives us nine-tenths of perception, it is the last of the five senses to come into activity.

Creative intellect is rare. Everyone cannot be an original thinker. The world's mental work is mainly done by a few matter-of-fact individuals. It requires peculiar geniuses of certain mental characters, an aptitude that qualifies a person for special success in a given line, one of distinctive taste, an inclination, a disposition and natural bent of intellect to originate and vizualize the telegraph, the telephone, the phonograph, the moving picture, the aeroplane and chiropractic. While everyone cannot be an original thinker, anyone can learn to be reliable, observe and husband the knowledge acquired by others, make it useful and profitable.

FUNCTION.

In physiology a function is a normal and specific action of any tissue, organ, or part of a living animal or plant, and is applied only to the action of an organ.

A function is a peculiar action of an organ which has a duty to perform. The performance of a physiological duty is a function. A physiological function is performed in obedience to a command.

An organ is a part of, or a definite structure of an animal or plant adapted to perform some specific function.

The action or actions of an organ are known as functions. A function may be expressed normally, or in too great a degree, or subnormal; a deviation either way from the standard creates conditions known as disease, is disease.

The functions include all of the vital phenomena of plants or animals, understood to be performed in a proper manner, unless otherwise stated. All functions are vital, directed by vital force, a force directed by an intelligence. Mechanical, thermal, chemical, electrical, magnetic, cohesion, gravity, centripetal and centrifugal forces differ from vital force which depends upon two original and independent elements, spirit and matter.

Vital force may be divided into neurism, nerve force, and bathism, growth force, energy. These two divisions of vital force are under the direction and control of individualized spirits. Phrenism, that force is of the mental, under the direction of the human will. Vital force is inherent in the organ or organism. Vital energy is the expression of vital force. Function is energy expressed by or through vital force. The actions which cause us to live are controlled by intelligences. Spirit is everywhere throughout the body. There are 144 brain centers from which spirit directs all the vital functions.

Functions are divided into animal and vegetative. The animal functions are those of the intellect, the voluntary motions. The vegetative relates to metabolism, anabolism (constructive m.) and catabolism (destructive m.). The vegetative function includes the unconscious, involuntary growing, or functionating after the manner of vegetables. The vegetative function is of the body; the cumulative is of the spirit. Either may be normal or abnormal. Bear in mind that a function is a duty to be performed, that behind the service there is an intelligence demanding a certain obligation, the performance of which is a function. These orders are known as impulses sent out over the communicative nervous system. Nerves carry motor impulses outward and sensational intelligence of the external requirements inward.

Physiology treats of the functions performed normally—in the usual manner. Functions which are pathological are performed in an unusual manner. Functions performed as desired are physiological. Innate is a director of the organic functions. Agents which cause an increase or decrease of functionating (disease) are from without, never from within.

Animal economy includes the laws which harmoniously govern an organization as a whole, man or animals. The functions of a human body, as a whole, are spoken of as the economic functions, the disposition and regulation of all the organs of the body. The organic functions are directed by spirit, as well in the new-born as in the educated adult.

Functions cannot be percented. We may speak of them in a comparative way, or a relative amount.

Function in physiology is applied to and refers to the action of an organ, or a part of an animal or plant. Function particularly refers to the special duty to be performed by an organ or parts.

Normal or proper functionating requires a normal condition of the nervous system; a condition, we will learn in our next lesson, depending upon a correct position of the osseous framework.

Science, we will learn in our last lesson of this course, is a systematized knowledge which enables us to demonstrate and assign to their place anything and everything known as phenomena which we can perceive with one or more of our senses; the science of functions include the accumulated knowledge of the qualities of the various functions of living tissue.

Functional activity refers to the physiological or pathological action of an organ.

Instead of examining the cells of dead tissue with a microscope for aberrant functions I have given my investigations to functional deviation in living tissue.

I want to repeat, in order to emphasize one of the physiological principles of chiropractic, that the performance of functions, normal or abnormal, depend upon the condition of the organ and the quality of innervating nervous tissue.

The vegetative function is that office in the human economy which controls the power of growing. It is concerned with nutrition and growth. In anatomy it refers to those organs and tissue which contribute to nutrition, the development and reproduction; those organs which have to do with the growth of the physical body. The processes of assimilation of nutritive material and its conversion into living substances is known as anabolism.

The cumulative function determines the quality of that which is accumulated by the mental, it corresponds in the spirit to the vegetative function in the physical. The quantity, character, peculiarity and the nature of the contents of the mental storehouse depends upon the condition of the physical; therefore, chiropractors knowing how to adjust the osseous system, the tension framework, have a normal and a religious duty to perform. As the vegetative function is subservient to the vital, so the cumulative is subordinate to the mental. It is to the spiritual body just what the vegetative function is to the physical body.

Normal functionating and normal temperature are co-existent, they constitute health. Disease is an alteration in tissue and function. The performance of functions above or below that of normal activity is due to the change in renitency, firmness and tension of the organ or part performing the act. Impulses delivered with normal force result in orders normally performed. Motive force exaggerated or decreased during the transit of an impulse over the nervous system results in conditions known as disease. The vegetative function depends upon the amount of vital force used in arousing latent energy. The quality and amount of mental impressions depend upon the cumulative function. Sane or insane ideas are the result of normal or abnormal perception. We receive impressions from the external world through the senses of touch, taste, smell, hearing and sight; qualities of the nervous system. We obtain knowledge, receive impressions, take cognizance of the existence and character of phenomena by means of sensation—molecular vibration of the nervous system. The force of sensations and impressions depend upon the condition of the nervous tissue.

A change in the structure or position of an organ creates over or under, too much or too little, function, a condition known as disease. There is a difference between ''disease is the result of over or under function'' and over or under function is disease. Functions performed normally is health, in an abnormal manner or amount is disease, a departure from a state of health.

Physiology treats of functions performed normally. Pathology discourses upon functions performed in an unusual manner.

The performance of functions depend upon the amount of energy stored and aroused by innervation.

Pathological physiology is the performance of functions by an excess or a deficiency of vital force.

Teratology is the science of abnormal growths, the result of vegetative functions performed in an abnormal and unusual amount.

All agents which cause increase or decrease of functionating (disease) are from without—could not be from the spirit—from within.

Vitality runs the vegetative function, while intellectuality directs the cumulative function. As the vegetative function may produce teratism, even so, the cumulative may accumulate monstrous intellectual conceptions. As we carry with us in this world perfect or imperfect bodies, just so, we take with us into the next world sane or insane ideas gathered in this world.

The cumulative function determines the contents of the intellectual storehouse. The condition of the physical determines the qualifications of the mental. We take with us into the beyond just what we have mentally gathered in this preparatory stage, whether those thoughts, impressions and recollections, are sane or insane, normal or monstrous, of reason or of a freakish mind.

VERTEBRAL ADJUSTING

The direct cause of disease (abnormal functionating and morbid tissue) is subluxated joints; about 95 per cent. of which are slightly displaced vertebrae; the balance will be found in other joints than those of the vertebral column. There are no nerves between the articulating surfaces of joints. Luxations of the toe joints cause corns and bunions.

A dorsal vertebra displaced ever so little, twisted out of its normal alignment, disarranges the costocentral, costovertebral, costo articulation, the juncture of the head of the rib with the body of the vertebra. A thoracic vertebra racked from its normal position affects the costotransverse joint, the articulation of the tuberosity of the rib with the transverse process of the vertebra. Its dislocation must of necessity displace the intervertebral articulation. The displaced bones of any luxated joint may impinge upon a nerve, or by their displacement cause a nerve to be stretched, thereby creating inflammation. A dislocated vertebra cannot do otherwise than displace two (cervical and lumbar), four (eleventh and twelfth dorsal) or six (the first to and including the tenth dorsal) articulations causing nerve tension.

Some authors on chiropractic state and use cuts to show how nerves are pinched because of occluded intervertebral foramina, the closing up of the foramina attributed to accidents or a settling together of vertebrae. These writers now use the word impingement instead of pinch, seeing the founder of chiropractic makes use of that term, yet they do not comprehend the difference between a nerve being impinged AGAINST and one pinched BETWEEN two harder substances. There are no intervertebral cartilage between the atlas and occiput and the atlas and axis, that by compression might narrow or occlude the intervertebral foramen. Atlas luxations are the cause of a large per cent. of diseases, which may be relieved by adjusting the displaced atlas. The displacement of other joints than those of the vertebral column cause nerve tension, a stretched condition; disease the result, and yet, no possibility of a nerve being pinched. I find that disease is caused by displaced vertebrae or other joints pressing against nerves; nerves are stretched because of displaced bones; the replacing of displaced portions of the neuroskeleton releases tension, consequently the conditions which cause disease are relieved.

The spinal cord does not entirely fill the vertebral canal. A wide space, or rather three spaces, intervene between its surface and the walls of the canal; this arrangement affords freedom of movement of the vertebral column without undue pressure or tension on the spinal cord. Two of these spaces are continued and surround the spinal nerves as they pass through the foramina affording the same freedom from pressure to the spinal nerves as is accorded to the spinal cord.

The difference in the height of a man at twenty-five and eighty, barring abnormal curvatures and luxations, considering the natural shortening or approximation of vertebrae, does not exceed one inch, usually less than half an inch. This shrinkage in height must be divided between the twenty-nine articulations from occiput to ankle. A slight bending of the neck of the femur should, also, be included. Vertebrae have epiphysial annular plates on the upper and lower surfaces of their bodies; each are developed from an ossifying center at the fifteenth to the twentieth year and join the body of the vertebra by the twenty-fifth year. These epiphysial plates are thickest at the circumference, gradually thinning toward the center. A vertebral column at or about the age of fifteen will show the various stages of fusion of the vertebral bodies and their surface plates. Bear in mind the distinction between the vertebral plates and the intervertebral fibro-cartilage discs; the cartilage of the former become ossified and eventually a part of the bodies, while the latter always remain cartilage. The point I wish to notice is that these epiphysial rings at the age of twenty-five are quite prominent; as age advances they approximate the height of the center of the intervertebral surface. Dividing this contraction of the vertebral column and limbs among all the articulations, it would average one-thirtieth of an inch. It should be also remembered that the spinal nerves become slightly contracted in length, firmer and narrowed in their diameter as age advances.

This slight difference mentioned in the length and diameter of the thirty-one pairs of nerves which arise from the spinal cord and pass out between the vertebrae, would fully make up the trivial variation found in the length of the spinal column and the size of the intervertebral foramina in adult and old age, as much so, as that found in the advancing stages of growth from infancy to adult age.

Kyphotic persons, known as hump-backs, will compare favorably, regarding health and longevity, with those who have not deformed backbones.

When we consider that the spinal cord is freely movable within the spinal canal and that the spinal nerves are afforded ample space for their emergence from the intervertebral foramina, we will see that normal movements do not compress the spinal cord or spinal nerves. The very slight difference in the size of the spinal foramina between the age of twenty-five and eighty would not be worth considering. Take into consideration the play, the amount of space between the occipital and the posterior arch of the atlas and the size of the nerves which pass out over the grooves, and between the atlas and the occiput there is no intervertebral cartilage, only a very thin hyaline, articular cartilage, which, if its thickness was shrunken to half, or if it was all absorbed, would make no appreciable difference in the size of the gap between the atlas and occiput, sufficient to compress or pinch a nerve—even if such were the case, would not the bending of the head forward ever so little relieve the compression by enlarging the gap?

Take your spinal column in hand. Do you not see that there is no intervertebral cartilage between the atlas and axis and the occipital bone and the first vetebra? Do you not see that the long, wide gap between the atlas and axis affords no possible chance for nerve compression—no more than there is between the atlas and occiput? If you think the first or second spinal nerves can be pinched, compressed or squeezed by the approximation of the atlas and the axis or the drawing together of the occiput and the atlas, just try to explain such a condition to your next prospective patient. The same kind of pressure that causes corns and bunions, and the many diseases which arise from impingement or a change in the amount of tension of the first and second pairs of cervical nerves, must also cause disease elsewhere. The rule must hold good throughout the body.

The filaments of nervous tissue create heat and transmit impulses, it is the only structure which can increase or decrease the amount of heat, increase or decrease the velocity of impulses or modify the force of reflex action, the bounding back of an impulse. Remember, the amount of function depends upon the renitency, the impulsive force obtained by the bounding back. Ease and disease depend upon the condition of nerves. Nerves furnish innervation and heat to all parts of the body, whether in normal amount, or more or less than normal. The organs of the body perform their functions normally when nerves are at ease and vice versa.

Center Place and Second Center Place.

Pathologists tell us that hemiplegia is "Usually due to cerebral disease." "The condition is due to hemorrhage, embolism, or thrombosis." "An escape of blood into one side of the brain arrests the action of this organ, so that the part of the body which is moved by nervous influence of this side of the brain is paralyzed." "Due usually to a lesion of some part of the corpus striatum and internal capsule, of the crus cerebri, or of the cortex or subcortex of the opposite side of the brain." A. P. Davis "Claims that osteopathic treatment offers better results than can be derived from any other source known, for the reason that blood (arterial blood to the parts) is the only tissue builder and preserver."

One of my earliest discoveries was that hemiplegia, paralysis of the lateral half of the body, was due to a displaced sixth dorsal vertebra; that displacements of the articulations caused extreme nerve tension; that by replacing the luxated vertebra, the nerve, or rather the fibers of the sixth dorsal nerve, resumed normal tension and normal functionating. In some cases it is alternate, one-half of the body and the opposite of the face, or it may affect the lower limb on one side and the upper limb on the opposite side. If the paralysis does not include the face and head, but the balance of the body, look to the cervical. In facial hemiplegia, paralysis of one-half of the face, look to the cervical. Infantile hemiplegia, birth paralysis, look to C. P. Hemirheumatism, affecting a lateral half of the body, look to C. P. Paralysis and rheumatism are opposite conditions; one exhibits too much function and the other a lack of action and sensation.

Adjust center place for diseases which affect the whole body, or a lateral half.

Knowing the region of dislocation, it is easy to locate the displacement and the affected nerve by noting the contour of the spinous processes and nerve sensation by palpation.

The ganglionic nerve-chains extend from the occiput to the coccyx; fibers of which extend into the cranium and become a part of one or more of the cranial nerves. The double axial vertebral nerve chains are distributing agencies for the nerves of organic life. They control the circulation of the blood, respiration, nutrition and all the vital processes. They are the involuntary nerves, not directly under the control of the human will. They are connected by communicating nerves, one with the other, and with the various organs, blood vessels and viscera.

There are many diseases which are caused by a displacement of the sixth dorsal vertebra. To illustrate, typhoid fever is the result of decaying animal and vegetable effluvia, a subtle emanation of a noxious, mor-

51

bific character, having an injurious influence on human beings when inhaled.   Poisons act on and contract the nervous system, contracted
nerves act on muscles pulling vertebrae out of alignment; vertebrae out
of alignment stretch nerves, cause increased contraction, vibration
and heat; excessive heat causes necrosis in those organs or parts to which
the fibers of the sixth dorsal nerves end in and innervate. Local inflammatory conditions occur, such as necrosis and supperation of the intestines, lungs, spleen, liver and degenerative changes in the kidneys.
The vertebral ganglionic chains distribute fibers to various parts of the
body, carry involuntary impulses, whether normal or abnormal, create
functions which result in health or disease.

To use the language of pathologists, ''The system reacts in some
way, as yet unknown, to check its progress and to bring it to a termination at the end of four weeks.'' ''It is impossible to cut short the
disease.''   ₁

In some cases the symptoms of typhoid continue for months or years.
This unlimited condition is known as ambulating or walking typhoid.

Cretinism appears during the first three years of life. It is a condition of physical, mental degeneracy and non-development. It is characterized by goitre, or an absence of the thyroid gland, premature ossification of bones, deformity of the head and face, large thick lips, pro-
truding tongue, misshapen cranium, lack of sensibility, stupid counte-
nance, thick neck, shortness of arms and legs, prominent abdomen, im-
becility or idiocy, arrested bodily growth, mental development lacking—
dwarfed idiots.

The ''sympathetic nervous system is based upon superstition and
while in vogue now, will not be in fifty years. It is unknown to the
P. S. C. and is replaced with a direct brain cell-to-cell nerve connection.
We have said right along that the basis of the sympathetic nervous
system was wrong because we are taught that man has 129 ganglions
which are equivalent to 129 brains. When I saw there was no use for a
sympathetic nervous system, I threw it out, and then just had to put
something better in its place, so I discovered Direct Mental Impulse.''
Since D. D. Palmer ceased to be the editor of The Chiropractor, its pages
do not teach and its clinics do not make use of the sympathetic nervous
system, the cranial nerves, the accessory, or communicating, or recurrent
nerves.

A case of hemiplegia will illustrate the difference between the
''direct mental impulse'' theory discovered by B. J. Palmer and so
taught to his students and that of the nervous system found in man
alive and dead, and known by all anatomists. To reach each portion of
the body affected by hemiplegia by the ''direct method'' would require
the adjusting of a half-dozen or more vertebrae, as given by the ''combination of functions'' method. This form of paralysis is the result of

one displaced vertebra impinging upon one nerve and not a "combination of functions." Considering the ganglionic chain of the sympathetic nervous system, the impingement is only on one nerve, one bundle of nerve-fibers which are distributed to the parts affected by the sympathetic ganglia. These ganglia are relays in the pathways for the transmission of impulses from the regions in which they arise to the tissue in which they are distributed. Communication between the central nervous system and the sympathetic is established through both efferent and afferent fibers. All spinal nerves are joined by gray rami communicantes from the sympathetic trunk. Corresponding communications exist between the cranial nerves and the sympathetic, but these occur farther toward the periphery and in not so regular a manner as the communications between the spinal nerves and the sympathetic system. Through this ganglionic distributing agency the fibers of one nerve reach one half of the body. This impingement will be found at center-place. In the "direct system" the half-dozen or more places adjusted, none of which were displaced, will make displacements, if moved, cause impingement upon nerves and affections in the portion where they end.

A case of hemiplegia (lateral half paralysis) has just been presented to me. The patient received pseudo-adjusting from the hands of the originator of the "direct mental impulse" system at atlas, axis, 3d, 5th, 8th, 9th and 12th dorsals, also, on the 3d lumbar, in all 8 places, missing center place, the 6th dorsal. The "direct mental impulse" system is anything but direct.

See last paragraph on page 254 of The Adjuster.

THE NERVOUS SYSTEM

In biology, any part of the body having a special function is an organ.

In all organic beings there is a vital principle called nerve-force, nerve energy, nerve-impulse, or vital force.

The force of the vital and intellectual depend upon the condition of the nervous system for the amount of their expression.

In biology, a system consists of those organs which taken as a whole contribute toward one important complex vital function—those structures which are anatomically or functionally related. We have the human system, the whole bodily organism, the osseous s., the muscular s., the digestive s., glandular s., the vascular s., the nervous s., the cerebro-spinal s., the central s., the sympathetic s., the peripheral s., the ganglionic s.

The nervous tissue contained in the cranium is known as the encephalon or brain; it comprises the cerebrum, cerebellum, pons and medulla oblongata.

The medulla oblongata is the upward continuation of the spinal cord, the transition is at the lower level of the foramen magnum. The medulla is from three-fourths to an inch long. The first cervical nerve emerges from the vertebral canal between the occipital bone and the posterior arch of the atlas. The hypoglossal, the twelfth cranial nerve, arises from the medulla oblongata inside the ring of the foramen magnum. The spinal accessory portion of the vagus nerve, the eleventh spinal nerve, arises in the cervical region of the cord, sometimes as low down as the sixth cervical nerve, including filaments or rootlets from each cervical as it passes upward. It is the only nerve which finds a passage way through the large oval opening in the occipital bone.

The pons Varolii lies between the medulla oblongata and the fore and back brains. Pons means a bridge; Varolii is the name of the person who first wrote of this portion of the brain.

The cerebellum is the posterior brain mass lying behind the pons and medulla and beneath the posterior portion of the cerebrum. It consists of two lateral hemispheres united by a narrow middle portion.

The cerebrum forms the largest part of the encephalon. The two hemispheres are joined by the corpus collosum composed of nerve fibres by which every part of the cerebral hemispheres are connected with each other.

The spinal cord, the central nervous system, occupies the upper two-thirds of the vertebral canal. It extends from the foramen magnum to the lower border of the body of the first lumbar vertebra. It does not fill the entire vertebral canal in length or breadth.

Gray says the encephalon or brain is a complex organ in which resides the highest functions—consciousness, ideation, judgment, volition, and intellect—together with the centers of special sense and for the mechanisms of life (respiration and circulation), and the agent of the will. It specializes the manifestations of the intellect.

Consciousness, ideation, judgment, volition and will are of the intellect, the understanding, creations of the mind. It specializes the manifestations of the intellect. It particularizes the exhibitions of life, actions created by intelligence.

Feeling, sensation, the faculty of perceiving stimulus and consciousness are senses of education, "centers of special sense," therefore, of the mind.

"The mechanisms of life (respiration and circulation)" I would prefer to say, respiration and circulation are two of the requisites of life, two indispensables upon which intelligent action depends. Respiration and circulation are not controlled by the mind, are not intellectual faculties, their action is past our comprehension; they are under the guidance of a superior intelligence than that of man. In which of the seven divisions of the brain does the mind reside? In which of the seven does the functional creator exist; where is his throne from whence he rules the organism?

Gray tells us that the spinal cord is composed of grey and white substancees interlaced with minute fibrils, some of which serve as conducting paths between the brain centers and the spinal centers, that associating systems unite these conducting paths. He also states, "A purely anatomical examination fail to reveal the functional relations in the fibres."

Through the nervous system the intellectual receives all impressions and appreciation of the outer world. Nerve vibration is associated with consciousness. By and through it thon adapts itself to thon's environments.

The bodily functions control all physiological action. By and through the sympathetic portion of the nervous system life is maintained.

Through evolution the nervous system has undergone remarkable differentiation and specialization attaining its maximum as a dominant ruler in the human species; however, some of the animals and birds excel in some of the senses, for instance that of smell and direction.

Anatomists usually divide the nervous system into two divisions, the cerebro-spinal and the sympathetic. I prefer those of special sense and vegetative, the animal and organic. The intellectual controls the nerves of animal life, while the spiritual intelligence runs the nerves of organic life.

Each nerve is a cord or bundle of fibers, a sheath or covering containing filaments, each fiber or filament being a distinct route of inter-course of motor (mental) or sensory impulses from their origination to their destination. Nerve fibers do not inosculate or anastomose as do blood vessels. Read page 865, fifth paragraph, of Adjuster.

The spinal nerve just as it emerges from the intervertebral foramen, divides into four branches. The posterior primary division divides into an internal and external branch. The internal supplies the bones, joints and the muscles about them with innervation; it may or may not supply the skin overlying them.

The posterior primary division of the spinal nerve springs from the trunk immediately outside the intervertebral foramina, passes backward between the adjacent transverse processes. These divide and subdivide repeatedly, while the distribution to certain areas are more or less con-stant, they are very variable. No nerve, cutaneous or muscular, has a definite prescribed area of distribution. The meningeal or recurrent branches are very small and variable. They re-enter the vertebral canal through the intervertebral foramen and supply the membranes and blood vessels of the cord and the vertebral ligaments. The posterior division of the spinal nerve furnishes sympathetic fibers for distribution in the walls of blood vessels.

Sometimes there is an increase or a decrease in the number of the vertebrae in the vertebral column; in such cases there is a corresponding increase or decrease in the number of spinal nerves. The dorsal root of the first cervical or sub-occipital nerve in rare cases may be rudimentary or entirely absent. The first and second cervical nerves do not pass out-ward from the spinal canal through intervertebral foramina, but between the occipital bone and the posterior arch of the atlas and the dorsal arch of the atlas and the lamina of the axis. The thirty-first nerve is occasionally absent, there are sometimes one or two additional rudi-mentary caudal pairs of minute filaments below the thirty-first.

About seven-tenths of the body is fluid. The blood is about one-thirteenth of the weight of the human body.

Read for yourself in The Adjuster, at your leisure, pages 231, 323 to 330, third paragraph on 733 (make correction on page 733, last two lines of third paragraph, read in the dorsal and cervical from the opposite side in the lumbar—, and 805 and 806.

In the vertebrate animals, the nervous system consists of two divisions. One includes the brain, spinal cord, the cranial and spinal nerves. The other division is the sympathetic nervous system. The activities of the body are controlled by nerve centers, by means of fibers which extend to all parts of the body, there ending in the muscles. Those nerve fibers which originate in organs, receive and send sensations, are called sensory. Nerves which are connected with the central nervous system may be made up of fibers which bear messages from sense organs, in the skin or elsewhere, to the central nervous system, the sensory fibers, or to other fibers (the motor fibers) which carry impulses from the central nervous system to the outside. Some nerves are made up of both kinds of fibers, they are called mixed nerves.

The nervous system is twofold in its stimuli, that which is somatic, from the external world, concerned in animal life, the outward actions of animals, and that which is interested in the processes of nutrition and reproduction, the visceral, the excretory, the alimentary tract, the blood and lymph of the vascular system.

It is twofold in its activity; it receives stimuli which incites incentive action, and motor responses which respond in movements.

It is twofold regarding diseases, that which is somatic, pertaining to the body-walls, skin, muscles and skeleton, and that of the viscera of the four cavities. Of all those organs collectively which are of the same or similar tissue which especially contribute toward one of the important, complex, vital functions; the nervous system is the only one which is directly affected with disease, all others being indirectly acted upon by their connection with the nervous system.

The cerebro-spinal and the sympathetic systems are known as the voluntary and the involuntary. The former includes the nerves of animal life, while the latter performs the functions of organic life. Heat production depends upon the excitation of the nervous system—upon the amount of molecular vibration. Respiration, circulation and heat are essential to life. These functions are performed in proportion to the innervating force which, if excessive or deficient, disease or death is the result. Remember, disease is functions performed in an abnormal amount. Heat may become so intense as to soften, necrose nerve tissue, thereby cause a diminution of vibratory action, of which we will learn more in our future lessons. Read page 415 of Adjuster.

I have always stated and maintained that over or under functionating is disease, not "that disease is the result of over or under function." There is a vast difference between these two statements. Let me repeat, over or under functionating, change of structure and position of one or more organs when present constitute a condition known as disease. Normal functionating, normal structure and normal position of organs are always present in health. When the organs of the body are in normal position, their structure normal, their functions performed in normal amount, there is health.

Life is intelligent action. Absence of life is coexistent with the separation of intelligence and material, spirit and matter, followed by dissolution, disintegration, separation into its component parts of the material body. The intellectual portion known as spirit is eternal, always existed and always will. Material always was, its form has been subject to change, as much can be said of spirit.

Delafield and Pruden in their Text-Book of Physiology, page 413, state, "It is known that certain drugs (a drug is any substance used as medicine, internally or externally) introduced from without may induce fever. Exactly how these various substances act in the incitement of fever is unknown, explain that the nervous system may play an important role in these disturbances is indicated by the fact that more or less persistent elevations of temperature may follow puncture or hemorrhage in the corpus striatum or lesions of the bulb or certain other affections of the nervous system." Hemorrhage is caused by necrosis, softening of the vessel walls, the result of too much tenion of the nervi vasorum.

All vital action depends upon the condition of the nervous system for expression. This includes mental, motor and sensory.

Pain is sensation of nerves because of over tension, the swelling is really an enlargement diametrically of the nervous tissue, counterbalanced by contraction.

There are two intelligences in man, Innate and Educated, spirit and mind, the creator and the created. Either one can direct (Innate the involuntary and Educated the voluntary) the functions in normal force and amount, providing the lines (nerves) of communication are normal in their structure and qualities.

The cerebrospinal system and the sympathetic nerve system are intimately connected, the latter is derived from and dependent upon the former; it is especially concerned in the dissemination of innervation, nutrition and the functionating of the vegetative organs.

The voluntary nervous system includes the twelve pairs of cranial and the thirty-one pairs of spinal nerves, which Educated learns to control during life. The sympathetic gangliated chains have three pairs of cervical ganglia, ten to twelve pairs of thoracic, four lumbar and four or five sacral, all told 21 to 24 distributing centers.

The involuntary nervous system, the organic nervous system, the great sympathetic group, distributes its fibers to the organs of the four cavities, the cranium, chest, abdomen and pelvis. Some organs are supplied with nerve fibres from other sources than the sympathetic: for instance, the heart receives fibres from the vagus, spinal accessory and sympathetic.

There are three layers of muscles in the back. The superficial, the deep facia and the trapezius. The deep facia is a dense fibrous layer attached to the occipital bone, the spines of the vertebrae, the crest of the ilium and the spine of the scapula. The trapezius muscle is attached to the external occipital protuberance, the spinous process of the seventh cervical and the spinous processes of all the thoracic vertebrae. To the atlas are attached nine pairs of muscles. To the axis are attached eleven pairs. To the remaining vertebrae are attached thirty-five pairs and a single muscle.

One of the functions of the nervous system is sensation, by means of which we keep in touch with our surroundings. Nerves connect organs located in different parts of the body so they may act as a united and harmonious whole. One important function of the body is that of will, a provision for the creation of thought. By the way, the cultivation of correct thinking is of great importance to a chiropractor.

Neuritis, Arteritis and Rheumatism.

Diseases are classified (nosology) by pathologists according to the standpoint from which they are viewed. Hereditary, congenital and acquired. Infantile, adult and senile. Conformable to their origin, zymotic (malaria, small pox and typhoid), infectious (transmission without contact) and specific (s. remedy, s. medicine, s. disease, having a specific cause, as syphilis and the eruptive fevers). Agreeably to their manner of occurrence, sporadic (cholera and cretinism), endemic (belonging to a special part of the country), pandemic (affecting all persons of a city or country). Toxic (poison). Compatible to their lesions (organic, structural change and functional). Local, general and constitutional (hereditary, in consequence of inherent or acquired defects).

Neuritis, an inflammation of the fibers of the nerve. Arteritis, an inflammation of the nerves of blood vessels. While arteritis is known as inflammation of an artery, the inflammation is really confined to the nervi vasorum, the network of nerves which surrounds a blood vessel. Rheumatism, an inflammation of the nerves of a joint. Medical authors class rheumatism among the self-limited affections, for which they give many probable causes.

Spinal nerves, see The Adjuster, page 515.

Neuritis and neuralgia, as conditions, are closely related. The former refers to the inflammatory condition, and the latter to the pain.

' The walls of arteries and veins are composed of a fibrilated sheath and three coats. The vasa vasorum, blood vessels of the blood vessels, enter the external coats, from which branches enter the middle coat, but not the internal. The blood is returned from the walls of the vessels by small veins, venae vasorum. The blood vessel walls are covered and permeated with a plexus, a network of nerves, the nervi vasorum. See Gray's Anatomy, page 577.

Arteritis is an inflammation of an artery, really an inflammation of the nervi vasorum. The inflammation may be in any one or more of the coats which form the vascular walls of arteries and veins. Arteritis obliterans, the closure or obliteration of the lumen of a blood vessel. Arteritis deformans, changes in the walls of blood vessels due to inflammation. Softening, calcification, fatty degeneration, abscesses, ruptures, hemorrhages, ulceration, infiltration between the coats of the artery, are because of inflammation of the nervi vasorum.

Inflammation (excessive heat) causes the vascular wall to become necrosed, softer than usual. Arterio-sclerosis may be pathological or physiological, as determined by age.

High tension and rapid pulse may be physiological or pathological.

Inflammation modifies physiological processes. Physiological functions pathologically performed are exaggerated or perverted capacities of the structure involved. Hemorrhage of blood vessels, excessive exudation of fluid through their walls is but a physiological process, the emigration of corpuscles, exaggerated.

Rheumatism may be acute or chronic, the former is characteristized by inflammation, fever, perspiration, pain and swelling of the joints. The latter is slow in progress, the fibrous structure of the joints are thickened and contracted. The fibers of the body affected may be that of nerves, muscles or tendons. Rheumatism is attended with loss of motion and often more or less deformity.

Gout is a form of rheumatism, more especially of the toes.

Gonorrheal rheumatism is the result of gonorrheal poison contracting nerves, drawing the second lumbar vertebra out of alignment. This displaced vertebra impinges upon nerves, causing nerve tension, continues the eurethral and rheumatic inflammation. Gonorrhea is often complicated with prostitis, inflammation of the prostate gland, cystitis, i. of the bladder, ephidymitis, i. of the upper part of the testicles, salpingitis, i. of the fallopian tube and other pelvic diseases. These accompanying ailments are because of displacements of lumbar vertebrae brought about by reflex action, an involuntary nerve contraction, the result of neuritis (inflammation of a nerve). Nerve and muscle contraction draw vertebrae out of alignment. Adjust the first, second or third lumbar vertebra.

Acute rheumatism should be relieved by one adjustment. In such cases, how about uric acid and bacteria as causes? Gorby.

Inflammation may be known by redness, enlargement, excessive heat and sensitiveness to pressure. An inflamed nerve may be recognized, when subcutaneous, by its hardened condition, its sensitiveness to pressure and its enlarged diameter. It is contracted lengthwise and enlarged diametrically. Knowing these conditions we are able to trace the pathway of subcutaneous nerves by palpation.

Neurology is the science which treats of nerves and their disorder. Nerves which are abnormal in their structure create abnormally performed functions, possess a greater or a lesser amount of heat than normal, their carrying capacity of impulses is above or below normal because of increased or decreased vibration.

A neurologist is one versed in the anatomy of nerves, their physiological and pathological functions—normal and abnormal action.

Read last paragraph, page 147 of The Adjuster.

Neuralgia has many prefixes, such as mammary n., intercostal n., degenerative n., sciatic n., idiopathic n. and stump n. Sometimes after an operation or an amputation, the stump of the subcutaneous portion covered by the scar and the portion amputated become the seat of neuralgic pains, which may render life miserable. The wearing of an artificial limb is sometimes impossible, as light pressure against the stump will produce severe pain, owing to the sensitive condition of nerves. These conditions may be relieved by adjusting the displaced vertebrae which impinge against the nerves. The same pressure which caused the pain before amputation is yet pressing upon the same nerves, therefore a true neuritis continues. The severed ends of the nerves may become bulbous, neuromata. This diseased condition is known as amputation neuroma. As the nerve is composed of many fibers there may be multiple neuromata. Amputation neuromata are composed of proliferated nerve-fibers turned upon themselves and imbedded in a dense fibrous growth.

Read pages 472 and 473 of The Adjuster.

The walls of an artery consist of a sheath and three coats. The inflammation may be confined to any one or more of these coverings which are known as the external, middle and internal coats. The walls of the blood vessels are permeated with a plexus of nerves. The vaso-motor nerves are of two kinds, constrictor and dilator, contracting and expanding. In health these have normal temperature, normal tension. In disease, there is either too much or a lack of tightness. Arteritis is the result of too much tension. Anemia is the result of not enough stretch.

Rheumatism is recognized by an inflamed, painful, swelled condition of one or more joints, i. e., the surrounding tissue of a joint. Rheumatism is neuritis of the joint nerves.

In neuritis, inflammation of nerves, the heat may be so intense, as to cause degeneration (softening) of nerve tissue, necrosis; the nerve tissue may even disappear entirely.

A temperature above ninety-nine is known as fever, its origin being a local inflammation—heat diffused through the nervous tissue.

When rheumatism is general look to e. p., when of one or both arms look to the dorsal. If of the lower limbs or lumbar region, the displaced vertebrae will be found in the lumbar, the lower the affection in the limbs, the lower the cause in the lumbar.

FEVER.

The medical profession are not agreed as to the cause, injuries or benefits derived from inflammation and fever.

Stengel's Text-Book of Pathology, date 1907, on pages 45 and 47, under the head of Nature of Fever, says, "These processes of heat-production and heat-dissipation are regulated in an orderly manner under the influence of the nervous system. Special centers for the production, dissipation, and regulation of heat have been described by the physiologists, though their location and method of operation still remain in doubt. Whatever the exact mechanism may be found to be, it is quite certain that in some way the nervous system exercises a control over production and discharge of heat.

"While fever occasions many disturbances and leads to various pathological consequences, it is not improbable that there is a certain measure of usefulness, in it."

McFarland states, "Inflammation is the sum of phenomena manifested by an injured tissue. The phenomena are, for the most part, reactionary and reparative; some are destructive and disintegrative.

"A careful analysis of the phenomena of inflammation leads us to the broad generalization that they are conservative in tendency, benign in disposition, and evidently the result of a carefully adjusted protective mechanism."

A. P. Davis in Neuropathy affirms, "The causes of fever are a mooted question. Many theories are advocated, but the most plausible seems to be that of central disturbance near the corpus striatum, due to blood pressure. The cause of the blood pressure is as much a mooted question as the cause of fever."

The Los Angeles Herald of May 27, 1912, reports, "It was expected that a crisis in the fever from which he has been suffering for seven weeks would be reached tonight. His temperature is 105 degrees. Physicians remained at his bedside throughout the night."

The production of animal heat is no more a process, a series of actions, than the heat created in a nail by a quick extraction from a piece of hard wood in which it had been driven. In animals and vegetation the temperature is increased by a greater atomic action, while in inanimate substances the heat is increased by a greater molecular vibration. Heat production in the animal economy is created by the vibration of molecules of which nerves are composed. It is a biological fact that nerves vibrate in proportion to the amount of tension. There is no special center for heat production, regulation and dissipation. Heat is a function of the whole nervous system, a discovery made by D. D. Palmer on July 1, 1903.

Fever is a symptom, it is associated with pathological conditions. Fever is not a disturber of functions; it, of itself, is excessive heat, diffused throughout the body, however, it is always concomitant with actions which are performed in too great a degree.

The quantity of heat is "regulated" by the amount of nerve-vibration. The "orderly manner" is determined by nerve tension. "The influence (power) of the nervous system" to produce heat in normal quantity depends upon the ability of the creator of life to transmit nervous impulses from a ganglionic center (Gould), known to physiologists as nervous influence, nervous energy, nervous force and nerve stimulus. The tissue of the nerve itself does not furnish the energy or the force. The impulses, the incitement of the mind or spirit (Webster), the influence of suggestion or prompting, furnishes a stimulus which arouses energy or force for the performance of functional acts.

Instead of the nervous system "exercising a control over the production of discharge of heat," the animal-tissue (the nervous system) is controlled by an intelligence known as spirit. Intelligence produces the actions which constitute life by animating the material body.

The "usefulness" of fever is made manifest by M. D.'s while sitting at the bedside of the patient, waiting and watching for the crisis of fever.

Dr. Davis in his brief statement above wisely sums up the opinions and conclusions of the medical profession regarding fever.

The word mechanism is mentioned twice in the above quotations. Webster defines mechanism as the arrangement or relation of the parts of a machine. Man, animal brutes and vegetables possess life, vital force, are not machines.

Dorland's Dictionary gives 100 kinds of fever and Gould's 150.

Fever is a condition in which the bodily temperature is elevated above the normal. The pulse is accelerated, its movement increased, there is general derangement of functions, thirst and loss of appetite.

Thirst, a desire to drink because of dryness, because of an inflammation of the mucous membranes of the mouth, fauces, pharynx, esophagus and stomach. Excessive heat dries and thickens the mucus of the mucous membranes, water is cooling and moistens the mucus.

Fevers are said to be symptomatic when functions are performed in an abnormal manner, producing vital phenomena not in accord with those of health—recognized by signs and symptoms. Signs of disease may be objective, apparent to the observer by examination, and subjective, when known only by the patient. Signs include auscultation, percussion, commemorative (those preceding the disease), diagnostic (those which accompany it and reveal the nature and seat of the disease), prognostic when they indicate its probable duration and termination. Fevers are essential when general, not depending on any local affection. Idiopathic when they arise without any known cause. Self-limited when they run a definite course under any and all treatment, and terminate in health or in death.

Surrounding temperature makes no difference in the temperature of the body. The body does not depend upon external heat for its temperature, but, upon nerve tension. Esquimaux often experience 60 to 80 degrees below zero. Equatorial countries endure 130 degrees above, making a variation of 210 degrees. The heat in oceanic steamers often 150 degrees. Some persons take Turkish baths which by frequent exposures are brought to the boiling point. Persons have lived for a few minutes in rooms wherein the temperature was 211. The "Salamander" withstood for 14 minutes a temperature of 338 degrees. His pulse on entering was 76, on coming out 130, yet there was no variation of bodily temperature. While the pulse varies, more or less, with the change of bodily temperature, exercise and mental agitation, but it does not accord with animal heat.

A rise of 2 or 3 degrees in the aged is more alarming than in the youth. As age advances nerve-tissue is less elastic, firmer, less yielding, not so pliable, does not so readily adapt itself to heat modifications.

Fever may be the result of traumatism or poisons. Nerves excited cause hyperthermia. Heat is a function of nerves—not of blood.

Rheumatism may be from trauma or poison. Gonorrhea is a direct effect from poison, while gonorrheal rheumatism is indirect, the poison causes nerve contraction, nerve tension draws vertebrae out of alignment; vertebrae awry stretch nerves, the effect of which we name rheumatism.

The pulse in scarlatina is more rapid, in typhoid fever slower. Some poisons excite, while others depress. In scarlatina the poison excites, in typhoid it depresses. This difference is owing to the nature of the poison ingested, injected or inhaled.

Delafield and Pruden in their work on pathology state, "Inflammation is a modification of physiological processes." They should have said, inflammation modifies physiological processes and the general temperature of the body.

Fever is destructive, not conservative.

In fever anabolism is decreased and catabolism increased.

The normal temperature of the body is about 98.5, although it drops almost two degrees after we have gone to sleep. It is ordinarily the highest at 5 p. m. because of labor, and the lowest at 4 a. m. on account of relaxation. The body temperature may be two or three degrees higher during violent exercise owing to nerve excitation. Bodily temperature depends upon nerve innervation, nerve excitation, not blood circulation.

Bodily heat may be increased by exercise, electricity, poisons, pressure on nerves and an undue amount of tension. Mechanical action excites, feet and hands are warmed by friction, temperature is increased because of nerve excitation. The chafing of nerves excite greater action, while blood circulation and its temperature remains the same. Masseurs, osteopaths and spondylotherapists, who rub, stroke, knead and tap the superficial soft parts of the body with the hand or an instrument for remedial purposes, excite or depress the action and functions of the nervous tissue, increasing or lessening nerve vibration, consequently, changing the temperature of the body. Operations are followed by a rise of temperature because of injury to the nervous tissue. Electricity stimulates, because of greater nerve tension. Poisons create more or less contraction of nerve tissue. Impingements excite, create greater tension. Nerve injuries produce excessive heat, consequently, pathological conditions.

We may have healthy (physiological) changes of temperature during the healing of wounds and fractures of bones.

In neuralgia there is no fever, no constitutional disturbance. Why! In neuritis the tension and pain is in the whole length of the nerve, while in rheumatism and many other diseases the stretch, the tension, is confined to a very short portion of a nerve.

Acute and chronic are antithetical terms; when applied to disease they refer to the duration. A disease is said to be acute when it is severe, of short duration, attended with danger, of rapid progress and its termination for better or worse is quickly reached. Chronic diseases progress slowly and are of long duration. Acute diseases should not become chronic and will not if the displaced portion of the neuroskeleton is properly adjusted.

Brain fever is diffused heat from an inflamed cerebrum or cerebellum or their membranes. Pneumonia, pneumonitis, is an inflammation of the lungs, when its diffused heat is spoken of it is referred to as lung fever. Pleurisy is an inflammation of the pleura, a serous membrane which covers the walls and viscera of the thoracic cavity. The exudation which collects upon its surface or in its cavity is the thickened viscid liquid serous secretion of the pleura. These diseases are acute, each should be relieved by one adjustment, one thrust upon the vertebra which is imping-ing upon the nerve whose fibers ramify the portion affected. In diseases of only a few days' duration, the vertebra does not become ill-shapened. In chronic diseases, those of long standing, the vertebrae become wedge-shaped; such require much time to reshapen back to normal.

Constipation and Costiveness.

Standard dictionaries use these two terms as synonyms, meaning nearly one and the same. Medical dictionaries make only a slight difference. In the practice of chiropractic there is a vast difference; this discrimination should be duly considered. Chiropractors should make a special distinction between constipation and costiveness. The two conditions resemble each other in the infrequency of evacuation, in no other sign or symptom are they alike. In the character of the stool there is a great difference. In costiveness the feces are scanty, dry, hard, compact and in chunks, yet the color is normal; the fluids from the spleen, pancreas, liver and intestine give it the normal color. In constipation the character of the stool may be normal; the sluggish movement of the feces may be owing to atony, a lack of tone or tension, or a relaxed condition of the bowels, or the organs of the abdomen may be flacid, weak and displaced.

The prolapsed condition of the stomach, kidneys, uterus, bowels, rectum, the conditions known as hernia, floating kidneys, prolapus uteri, and hemorrhoids are because of a lack of tone, a relaxation of the abdominal nerves. Chiropractors should become aware of this condition resulting from relaxation and undue tension.

Constipation is due to functional inactivity of the intestinal canal, or from a lack of biliary, pancreatic and other secretions; obstructions of the intestinal canal, or paresis, paralysis of the intestinal walls, or the use of certain food or drugs, or a general depression of vital activity. Each of these when known will suggest to a chiropractor the change of injecta necessary and the proper adjustment—not adjustments. In constipation there is a lack of vermicular or muscular motion, waves of alternate circular contraction and relaxation of the intestinal tube by which the contents are propelled onward, as is the circulation of the blood by the nervi vasorum.

There is a condition known as reversed peristalsis, in which the waves of contraction and relaxation are reversed, the contents of the intestinal tract, or a portion of it is reversed and thrown backward. When the bile is furnished in an unusual quantity it is thrown upward and into the stomach, and from thence it is ejected through the mouth. In peristaltic unrest the bowels are in a state of abnormal mobility, the evacuations too frequent. The lesion should be located and the over-tense nerves restored to their normal tonicity.

Coarse food, such as corn meal and graham, increases the vermicular motion, because of its action, excitation by chafing of the nervous tissue of the intestine, whereas, white flour does not excite, it is smooth and pasty.

67

Costiveness is accounted for by a lack of moisture; the kidneys are too active, they secrete and excrete more than their usual quantity of fluid, thereby robbing the stool tract of its normal amount of moisture. Bear in mind that costiveness is because of a k. p. luxation and constipation is not. In costiveness adjust the 12th dorsal, for by its displacement the distance between its inferior articulating processes and those of the first lumbar are increased, thereby stretching the nerves which innervate the kidneys. Tense nerves, like stretched wires of a musical instrument, increases vibration, excitement and heat, a condition known as inflammation. Constipation and costiveness are two entirely, distinctly different conditions.

Bones have a normal limit in their movement—I refer to the mobility of joints, the articulations, the places of union between two or more bones—more than normal is abnormal, pathological.

How do I diagnose, determine the nature of the case and know where to adjust? This is done in far less time than it takes to describe the diagnostication, and much more comprehensive were you to see it performed. For the class a few cases demonstrated is worth more than any number not shown or proven. For example, a case is presented for class benefit. An ingrown toe nail, a callus on the plantar surface, soft and hard corns. I may say to you that the ingrown toe nail is because of a lumbar luxation, the soft and hard corns are from slightly displaced joints, that is, the articular surfaces of the toe joints are subluxated the same as in the joints of the vertebral column. These displaced bones, whether in the joints of the toes or the vertebral column, stretch nerves which are attached to the surfaces of those bones, or to be more definite, the nerves are attached to muscles which are secured to bones by tendons, tension creates conditions known as disease. There are no foramina in the toe joints, and those in the spine, together with the long gaps between the occiput and atlas and the atlas and axis, have nothing whatever to do with the tension of the spinal nerves and their branches. The hard and soft corns are the same, except that a soft corn is between the toes and is kept soft by moisture. The foot has seven tarsal bones and the hand has eight carpal bones. The callus on the bottom of the foot is because of a displaced tarsal bone, or at the articulation of the tarsal and metatarsal bones. To demonstrate that the callus on the plantar surface was because of a subluxated tarsal bone, that the corn was from a slightly displaced toe joint and the ingrown toe nail came from a lumbar luxation I would make the adjustment for each at different clinical lectures, but for a private practice I would adjust all three ailments at the same call.

Cordelia, Risley, and Mrs. Kale).

It is well to know of the construction of the parts we are handling. This branch of knowledge is known as anatomy. We should be acquainted with the vital processes of animal organisms—physiology. It is necessary that we should be acquainted with material and vital changes known as diseases—pathology. We ought to know specifically of the cause of disease as comprehended by chiropractors—etiology. The nature of the disease should be known—diagnosis. About one chiropractor in a hundred can give a definition of these terms and make intelligent use of that knowledge. However, I would rather have you comprehend one idea than to learn a dozen you do not understand.

How do I diagnose? First: I make use of clinical diagnosis. I study the signs of disease as exhibited by outward appearance which indicate a certain disease or morbid condition, also, the symptoms as related by the patient, who usually considers all cases where the evacuation of the bowels are infrequent, or incomplete, more or less fecal matter retained in the intestine, as constipation. As I question the patient I bring in differential diagnosis, by which I determine whether the condition is one of constipation or costiveness. Then the diagnosis of exclusion is made use of. There may be symptoms which might belong to and be associated with other diseases; these I exclude, leaving only one or more symptoms or signs which unerringly point to a certain vertebral luxation. Very few chiropractors make use of differential diagnosis; in fact not one in a hundred chiropractors make any diagnosis at all, have no use for physiology, pathology, anatomy, symptomatology, orthopedy or etiology. We ought to so conduct our exercises that each student wuld see the utility of being acquainted with these branches.

If I determine that I have a case of costiveness, of which the larger share of those who consider themselves suffering from constipation are; to assure myself and the patient that I am correct I make use of physical diagnosis. I palpate the spine in order to locate the 12th dorsal vertebra. The region of the 12th dorsal is readily found by placing the thumb under the lower rib, the outstretched fingers will give you the location of the 12th dorsal, making an allowance for the difference in the height of your patient; in time you will do this unconsciously. Having located the 12th dorsal by the means spoken of and a certain rate of motion best adapted to determine such inequalities in the contour of the spine as are caused by slight or partial displacements, NOT A CLOSING TOGETHER, NOT AN OCCLUSION. A displacement displaces vertebrae, spreads them apart, does not draw them together. To close them up would not be displacing. To luxate, dislocate would not be to draw the bones more compactly together. I proceed to palpate on both sides of the spine, using one finger and thereby determine which one or both of the 12th pair of nerves and the one or both of the kidneys are affected. This is determined by the rigidity of the nerves; those affected will be swollen and sensitive to pressure. Palpation is made by a vertical movement back and forth of a half-inch. The sensitive, contracted nerve or nerves may be followed to the affected kidney or kidneys. This procedure is known as nerve-tracing, an art not known to pathologists, the subcutaneous nerves thusly followed are not known to anatomists. This diagnosis is of no value to the one who does not comprehend it or does not make use of it, to the one who adjusts anywhere and everywhere regardless of the determination of the nature of disease it is valueless, to the one who adjusts without making a scientific discrimination, it is worthless, to the one who adjusts every other vertebrae today and the intervening one tomorrow it would be despised, to the one who adjusts every vertebrae for any and all diseases, commencing at the atlas in order to drive the disease down and out it would be condemned. A student of the Bohemian thrust wrote me ''I lay awake at night searching the depths of my creative ability for a painless thrust. For the last three years I have clinked each vertebrae of the entire spine without pain or discomfort to the patient. With this thrust I cannot jump about here and there in the spine, but must start at the sacrum and end at the occiput, and I have the satisfaction of knowing that I have set every vertebrae where it belongs, plump against the facet of its neighbor.'' This method was called ''reconstruction of the spine for constitutional correction.'' This developer and discoverer had no use for specific, definite, scientific adjusting.

In chiropractic there is no need of a laboratorial diagnosis, whether made by chemical analysis, microscopical examination, or a bacteriological study of the discharges from the kidneys or bowels, they do not tell chiropractors anything of value. A laboratorial diagnosis is not chiropractic, it is allopathic—I say, examine the living for morbid or abnormal functions—you will not find them in the lifeless cadaver or the inert cast-off refuse. Normal urine is of a clear amber color. There should not be any deposit in the bottom of the vessel. One urination may show an off color or a deposit, and the next micturition look o. k.

An osteopath author says, ''Constipation is the cause of a large per cent of diseases. ''He should have said, Constipation is associated with a large number of diseases, and then in all probability nine-tenths of his constipation cases are those of costiveness.

One chiropractic author speaks of ''an analysis of the morbid substance'' of urine. He evidently has the same idea of urine as has another author of equal chiropractic intelligence who says, ''The poisons resulting from the constipation go through the body and cause this fevered condition.'' Morbid urine would be that which is diseased. Disease is functions. performed in a greater or a lesser amount than normal. What are the functions of urine? What are the physiological actions of the feces? In what organic system do you place the stool or urine? Why not talk and write on biology? Living tissue, only, exhibits functions, they alone have power to create health or disease. Feces and urine have no nervous tissue, they have no functions to perform. Poisons are not created within the body. That which has a deleterious effect on the nervous system is from without. All fevered conditions are because of diffused inflammation. The morbid process known as inflammation is the result of nerve tension. Nerve tension is because of trauma or toxine. The condition of constipation does not produce poison. . Poisons decrease or increase nerve action. Evacuation and micturition remove waste material. The organic waste products, the undigested residue of the food, epithelium, intestinal mucus and other waste material are not tissue, they do not assist in forming any definite structure of the body. It is difficult for some persons to clear their mentalities of the cobwebs of superstition.

In many diseases the evacuation of the bowels is not normal because of the constructive and assimilative changes known as anabolism and the retrograde and destructive processes of catabolism.

There has been much determined by chiropractors, yet there remains much more to be ascertained and defined by us with clearness concerning anatomy, physiology, pathology, symptomatology, etiology and diagnosis which is not in accord with noted authors on these subjects, also, some statements made by standard authors which we as chiropractors do not agree with. Were we to agree with the doctrines of allopaths, we would be allopathic. For allopaths to agree with us would be to make chiropractors of them. (Dr. Kulp).

Much has been written by medical men regarding spinal pathogenesis, the special origin or development of disease because of abnormalities of the spine, but it remained for chiropractors to demonstrate that such is a fact.

Trauma, Toxine and Auto-Suggestion.

Trauma singular, traumata plural, an injury or wound.

Traumatic of, or pertaining to, or due to a wound or injury.

Traumatism, the morbid condition of the system due to a trauma.

Trauma a noun, the name of a condition, the injury or wound which is the cause of a diseased condition.

Traumatic, an adjective, pertaining to a wound, or that which is caused by a wound, e. g., t. abscess, t. amputation, t. appendicitis, t. cataract, t. dislocation, t. fever, t. hemorrhage, t. inflammation, t. suggestion, t. lesion, t. disease, t. medicine and t. back.

Traumatology, a treatise on wounds, the science of injuries, a description of wounds and the disabilities arising therefrom.

Diseases which are caused by displaced osseous tissue or wounds are said to be traumatic or lesional. E. H. Laughlin in his ''Quiz on the Practice of Osteopathy'' makes frequent use of the word lesional in place of its synonym cause.

Toxin or toxine, means poison. Toxic is poisonous. Toxicology is the science (the knowledge) of poisons. A toxicoligist is one versed in poisons, one who knows the changes likely to be produced in functions by the use of drugs.

A poison is an animal, vegetable or mineral substance which, when introduced into the system as ingesta, by injection, inhalation, or external application, causes such changes in functions as to produce disease or death.

A chiropractor does with his hands just what an M. D. aims to do with drugs. An osteo aims to do with his hands that which an M. D. does with medicine.

Do not forget for one moment that all organic functions are the characteristic work of organs or an organism directed by an intelligence known as spirit. This intellectual being transmits its impulses, its commands, over the nervous system by molecular vibration.

Poisons are irritative, cause inflammation, excessive nerve vibration, or they may be sedative or narcotic, produce stupor, reduce vital power, produce slower vibration.

Modification of functions are known as disease.

Medical men divide poisons into two classes, organic and inorganic. The former includes those poisons supposed to be developed within the body and cause disease. The latter includes deleterious substances from minerals, plants and snake venom.

Toxine in biology, as understood by medical men, is a poisonous substance produced by microorganisms. Of these, two kinds are recognized,

72

animal toxine excreted by certain animal cells, and the poison produced by bacteria.

All nerve irritants are traumatic, lesional or of toxic origin; cause abnormal functionating, pathological action.

Toxicosis is a disease caused by poison, an abnormal condition of the nervous system.

A toxicide is a remedy, an antidote, an agent, used to destroy the effects of another poison, not as a chemical antidote, but because of its opposite effect on nerves.

Landois in Human Physiology says: "The apparent increase in the temperature of inflamed parts is by no means dependent upon increase in the temperature above that of the blood, a condition that has never been observed." In other words: the temperature of inflamed parts is not dependent upon nor coincident with an increased temperature of the blood. This condition, a rise in the temperature of the blood, corresponding to that of the inflamed organ or portion, has never been observed. Inflammation and fever are not subject to, are not influenced by, do not rely upon the quantity nor the temperature of the circulating fluid.

Within certain limits of intensity heat is essential to the development of all organized beings; above a certain degree, it is destructive to all organization and life.

At birth the temperature of the infant is slightly above that of the mother. During childhood the temperature gradually approximates that of the adult.

Heat production and heat regulation, maintaining the same constant bodily temperature regardless of the surrounding degree of cold or heat below or above that of the body, has been and is, a problem to the medical profession. Inflammation and fever, pathological heat conditions, do not offer to the germ theorist any solution of this perplexed question.

Howel's Text-Book of Physiology says: Anesthetics and narcotics such as ether, chloroform, cocain, chloral, phenol and alcohol, may be applied locally to a nerve and the conductivity and irritability lessened, or suspended entirely at that point, and restored when the narcotic is removed." Poisons affect nerves, not blood.

The following biological principles which go to make up chiropractic science should be known and made use of by practitioners.

Nerve fibers possess the property of conducting impulses outward and inward. The amount of impulsive force is determined by the rate of transmission, the rate of that action upon the quantity of vibration and the amount of that movement upon tension. Physiological and pathological activity between peripheral end-organs and their central connection is dependent upon nerve tension. The specific energy of a nerve is due to its anatomical structure, its elasticity and tension.

A nerve pressed upon by a fractured or luxated bone would be stretched were it not for the responsive principle of life which resists pressure. The impulsive force normally conveyed by the nerve is modified by the elastic resistance known as renitency. The result is either too much or not enough functionating, conditions known as disease. The contraction and expansion of the nervous system has a normal limit known as tone, the basis upon which I founded the science of chiropractic. Any deviation therefrom is recognized as disease. Tone denotes normal temperature, normal structure, normal tension and normal vibration of nerves.

An angle worm, when relaxed, may measure six inches. Press against it, impinge upon it, try to stretch it, and immediately a response of increased tension is observed; it contracts lengthwise and its diameter is increased. This ability of elastic resistance to any opposing force is an inherent quality of all living matter. Dead material does not possess it. An impingement upon a nerve calls into action two opposing forces. The impinging body tends to stretch the nerve, while the inherent principle of self-preservation exerts an activity toward contracting it.

Reflex action is the bounding back of an impulse; the conveyance of an impression from the central nervous system ,and its transmission back to the periphery through a motor nerve. The amount of function depends upon the renitency, the impulsive force obtained by the bounding back.

Traumatism, as the cause of disease, increasing or decreasing functionating, is direct by displacing osseous tissue. Auto-suggestion and poisons, as causes, are indirect. They draw vertebrae out of alignment by the contraction of nerves and muscles.

Insanity may be caused by auto-suggestion, continued thinking upon one subject without rest. In such cases the third cervical nerves will be found affected. Correct by adjusting the third cervical vertebra.

Whether or not a given substance should be included under the term drug depends upon the purpose for which it is sold (as regards the seller) or used (as regards the purchaser). Any substance or preparation used in treating disease is a drug. Medicine as defined by the medical profession includes any drug or remedy used in the treatment of disease. A remedy is defined as that which cures, paliates or prevents disease. In its broadest sense it is defined as the art or science of healing diseases, more especially the administration of internal remedies. Thusly defined, a drug refers to the solid or liquid used in the treatment of disease, while that of medicine includes the drug or remedy used, also, the study and ability to treat disease. Medicine is divided into internal and external, the former refers to the treatment of organic diseases, abnormal functions and abnormal tissue, while the latter refers to surgery, the treatment of external diseases.

In 1908 James Gillman, a rancher on Mount Hamilton, Cal., who had been insane for several years, was bitten by a rattlesnake on the hand. The hand became swollen and showed the usual symptoms of snake bite. A few hours later the effects of the venom was no longer visible, and Gillman was restored to saneness, his mind became as clear and active as it ever had been. The poisonous venom had acted as an antidote, its contractile quality upon the nervous system had drawn the displaced vertebra, which caused his insanity, into alignment, accomplishing just what the chiropractor would have done by hand.

Bacteria, microbes, or microorganisms are microscopical vegetation, or those minute animals visible only with the aid of the microscope which live and develop in fluids or on moist surfaces and multiply with great rapidity. They subsist on dead organic material, are parasitical scavengers.

Mould, a fungus, grows on decaying vegetable matter, such as bread, cheese, gum and ink. Lippincott's Medical Dictionary says of the two latter, ''Destroying their valuable properties.'' As much might be as wrongfully said of the mould on bread, cheese and stagnant pools of water. The fact is that putrifying animal matter invites living scavengers, whether buzzards or microbes; while decaying vegetables and motionless water make suitable conditions for the growth and multiplication of vegetable life.

Autosuggestion is suggesting to one's self. Nerves are the means, the channels of communication of one's own thoughts and very often those of another. That other may be in the physical, near or far distant, or an astral being existing as a spiritual intelligence.

Nerves need mental and physical rest.

All functions, every act of the body, voluntary and involuntary, are directed by and through impulses (thoughts) passed over the nerves, the means of communication.

CATARRH.

This term was originally applied to inflammation of the mucous membrane of the nasal and respiratory passages and known as a cold; it is now extended to the mucous membrane of the bronchial tubes, stomach, intestines, appendix, colon, bladder, uterus, urethra and vagina.

A mucous membrane is a thin tissue which lines the canals, cavities and the inside of hollow organs which communicate externally by different appertures. It is the inside cutaneous tissue, similar as is the outside skin; it has certain functions to perform, and subject to diseases as is the outside cuticle.

Mucous membranes secrete a mucus, viscid, gummy secretion, analogous to vegetable mucilage. It is albuminous, like the white of an egg.

The mucus preserves the membranes and keeps them moist, a condition suitable for the performance of their functions. The mucus coating on the mucous membrane of the stomach prevents the stomach from self-digestion.

Mucus is secreted and exuded through the membrane, a process known as osmoses, or dyalisis; it is exuded, not circulated.

Mucous membranes are well supplied with arteries, veins, lymphatics and nerves.

In the acute stage of inflammation, the mucous membrane is at first dry and swollen.

The catarrhal discharge is purulent, tenacious, thick and ropy or stringy. It is at first frothy, then spots of gummy pus. In color it is at first white, then yellow and finally green. In recovery, under adjustment, the discharge will become thinner and more plentiful for a time as it returns to its natural consistency.

Pathologists define catarrh as an inflammation of a mucous membrane. The thickening mucus is a result of a membrane being inflamed.

Catarrh may be acute or chronic.

Catarrh of the nasal mucous membrane is known as rhinitis.

Inflammation of the bronchial tubes results in bronchitis or pulmonary catarrh.

Hay fever is the result of the mucous membrane of the eyes and air passages being inflamed.

Asthma, suffocative catarrh, is the congestive swelling of the bronchial mucous membranes which narrows the lumen of the bronchial tubes.

Cystitis, inflammation of the bladder.

Gastritis, inflammation of the stomach.

Inflammation of the eustacian tube, catarrh of the ear, otitis.

Endocolitis, inflammation of the mucous membrane of the colon.

76

Enteritis, inflammation of the mucous membrane of the intestines.

Cervicitis, inflammation of the lining membrane of the neck of the uterus.

Inflammation of the mucous membrane of the uterus is known as metritis.

Epidemic catarrh, influenza, grip, is from a condition of the atmosphere.

Endoappendicitis, inflammation of the mucous membrane of the appendix.

Gonorrhea is venereal catarrh, inflammation of the urethral mucous membrane.

Menstruation is a periodic discharge of mucus from the surface of the mucous membrane of the uterus, together with an excretion of blood from the vascular vessels of the mucous membrane of the uterus. It is often accompanied by local and systemic changes. The hyperemic condition of the uterine blood vessels is owing to increased temperature. The finer blood vessels of the uterine mucosa rupture, allowing the blood to escape.

During the menstrual flow and the time in which physiological menstruation gradually ceases, the nervous system is excited, a physiological rise of temperature is experienced. Many diseases, or ailments, which are usually very slight, are greatly increased during the menstrual discharge and aggravated at the time of the change of life. As to the **why**, pathologists offer no explanation. During some diseases, such as typhoid or typhus fever, the menses disappear. Some poisons excite the nervous system, while others depress, diminish vital energy, lower nervous functional activity, causing muscular relaxation.

Catamenia is the name of a condition, the periodic menstrual discharge of mucus and blood from the uterus. The menses is the recurrent monthly excretion of mucus and blood during sexual life from the genital canal of the female. The amount of mucus and blood leakage depends upon the degree of inflammation.

Menstruation is an organic function controlled by an intelligence, and not of the mind or mental. This periodic action responds to the solar or lunar month of 28 days, not the man-made calendar month of 30 days. It is said that most women menstruate during the first quarter of the moon and only a few at the time of the new or full moon.

The menopause, the grand climacteric, is the change or turn of life, the natural cessation of menstruation.

Puberty and the menopause denote climacteric periods, during which the physical, mental, and moral nature of the female is taxed more than ordinarily. All affections are intensified; some diseases are manifest at these periods which before or after were latent, or at least apparent only in a mild form. The cause lies not in the disturbance of the blood, it is not a process of purification, nor is it for the purpose of removing an excess of nutriment from the body. It is the physical condition resultant from increased nerve tension. Menstruation is a function, the performance of which, normal or abnormal, depends upon the condition of the nervous system; its cessation is as natural as its appearance.

Many ailments, not of the generative organs, are intensified at the climacteric periods. They are no more dependent upon the condition of the uterus than dysmenorrhea, hysteria, chlorosis or hysteralgia. At these periods the nervous system becomes more tense, thereby intensifying conditions known as disease.

The uterine mucosa (the mucous membrane) is inflamed and swollen at each monthly period. This is the actual source of the hemorrhage known as menses. Preceding the hemorrhage and immediately after, there is a mucoid excretion, which at other times would be known as catarrhal discharge. Chronic inflammation of the uterine mucosa may result in a discharge of portions of the mucous membrane, the resultant of excessive heat, necrosis.

The theory of some physiologists is that the inflammation of the uterine mucosa is for the purpose of creating a raw surface upon which the ovum may be readily grafted, aiding it in becoming attached to the maternal organism as a parasite upon its host. Greater nerve tension creates an increase in functional activity. The philosophy of this phenomena is readily comprehended when we take into consideration the extreme sensitiveness of the female during these climacteric periods. The senses of smell, taste, sight and hearing are more acute than ordinary. These conditions abnormally expressed, are by no means resultant from the change, but because of greater nerve tension.

Any disease arising at puberty or the menopause should be adjusted for, just the same as though appearing at any other time.

Vicarious menstruation is the menstrual flow from some part or organ other than the vagina. The above knowledge and philosophy accounts for what is known as compensatory menstruation.

Vicarious, compensatory, a substitute, taking the place of another, the assuming of a function belonging to another organ. V. respiration, an increased respiratory action in one lung to make up for the diminished action of the other. V. secretion and excretion may be increased in one part of the body instead of the usual function in another. V. diarrhea, an increased discharge of watery stool due to inaction of the kidneys, known as compensatory diarrhea. V. menstruation, a periodical bloody discharge from the stomach, nose, breasts, rectum, the pores of the skin or other parts of the body, occurring at the time of, and taking the place of, in part or whole of the menses.

Blood-sweating, a bloody discharge from the pores of the skin is considered vicarious when present in absent menstruation. It is an effect from a nervous disorder. Blood corpuscles have been found in the escaping drops of red sweat. Yellow fever at times is attended with bloody sweats. Biliary pigment has been found in the sweat of jaundiced persons.

You will find a brief description of, and where to adjust for, the above diseases in the Adjuster. I prefer to give you some ideas of value not found in the Science, Art and Philosophy of Chiropractic. These lectures are intended as an appendix to the Adjuster, not a Mail Course, not a Correspondence Course, nor a Post Graduate Course.

IMPULSE.

In our last lesson we learned that intuition is a knowing without reasoning. That instinct is a natural inherited impulse, unassisted by reasoning.

An impulse is a spontaneous incitement arising from the feelings of the mind or spirit in the form of an abrupt and vivid suggestion prompting some premeditated action. An impulse suddenly starts or drives a thought forward to action.

Thoughts are entities; they exist, are created by imagination, reflection, mediation, judgment and reason; they are elaborated. They may be transferred from one intelligent being to another by signs, speech or telepathy. A sign is that which communicates an idea, speech consists of articulate sounds transferred by atmospheric vibration, telepathy is the communication of ideas between two minds at a distance from each other without the aid of words or signs.

The power or force of thought depends upon its momentum, and momentum upon the impetus received from nerve vibration during transmission. Vibrations receive their force from the amount of heat. The amount of molecular action and heat are coexistent. Molecular action decides the quantity of heat. Heat determines the amount of molecular action. The quantity of heat depends upon tension, and tension upon excitation. Normal stimulus is furnished by Innate, the spirit, a segment of Universal Intelligence. Too much or too little excitation, stimulation, is the result of over-tension. Over-tension from pressure, displacement of the tension frame (bones) and nerve toxication.

Morbid impulses are qualified and differentiated as animal, destructive, homicidal, suicidal, uncontrollable, and especially those of an insane character. An impulse denotes action, not an entity.

Function is the special and normal action of any organ or part of a living animal. This includes the natural action of any mental faculty. Pathological functions are those performed in a greater or lesser degree than normal.

Force is that power which produces or arrests motion, that which may be converted into motion, the rate of transforming energy.

Vitality is the vigorous active principle upon which individual life depends.

Vital force is that principle of life which imparts energy. It is inherent in each organ of an organism.

Energy is the internal, inherent power, the product of activity, that which is aroused by an impulse.

Nerve-vibration carries thoughts, commands, orders, known as impulses when in transit over the nervous system.

Thoughts gather force, receive impetus, while being transmitted, the amount depending upon the quantity of nerve-vibration.

Momentum is the force of motion acquired by the movement of thoughts, the impetus received from nerve-vibration.

Tone is the normal activity, strength and excitability of the various organs and functions as observed in health. Tone is a response of tonicity.

Tonicity is the normal elasticity of the filamentary or threadlike structures of the body, the nervous system.

To innervate is to supply with nerve-force. To enervate is to deprive of nerve-force.

An impulse is a communicated thought. Impulses are conveyed over the nervous system by means of vibration.

Thoughts originate in man, animal and spirit. They are forwarded by atmospheric and etheric vibration. In spoken language by the former and by the latter where the affections of one mind are acted upon by the thoughts or emotions of another without communication through the ordinary channels of sensation, viz., the five senses.

There are two kinds of impulses, sensational and motor. Motor impulses go outward and sensational inward. The motor is twofold, one originating in the mind of the physical, governs animal functions, the nerves of animal life, it is under the control of the human will; the other is not under the control of the human will but that of spirit, and controls the sympathetic nerves of organic life, creating and continuing an intellectual existence. A sensational impulse is one which comes from without, one which creates within us sense impressions of our environments.

sense impression is no more or less than a recognition of nerve vibration, which is set in motion by the force of a sensational impulse. An impulse (a thought in transit) may be passed from one intellect to another, as in hypnotism and telepathy, or it may be transported from one portion of the body to another. In the latter case the nervous system is the transmitting medium.

An impulse does not make a circuit. Mental, motor, impulses go away from the central nervous system. Sensory impulses go to the central nervous system and away from the external, and to the origination of nerves. Motor or sensory impulses do not make a circuit, they do not circulate. Motor impulses may be of the mental or spirit, the sensory is of the mental.

Life (intelligent action) is the response to an impulse. This is true of the voluntary and involuntary functions. The former are those of the human will, the latter are those of the spirit. The impulse in transit is the thought sent out, it always remains the same in its requirement and command; however, its force may be augmented or decreased, owing to the amount of nerve vibration.

Functions performed normally, with normal force, produce activity known as health. Functions performed with more or less force than those indicating health is disease. Either of these conditions is life, one of health and the other of disease.

Pathology is modified physiology. Pathological operations are physiological acts modified. Processes which are pathological are but modified functional movements. Physiological impulses may become pathological in their expression.

The spiritual or organic impulses are transmitted over the sympathetic ganglionic nervous system, the nerves of organic life which ramify the viscera of the four cavities of the body, whereas the mental impulses are of the mind, under the control of the human will; they go to the somatic portion of the body over the anterior and posterior branches of the spinal nerves. It will be seen that the impulses of spirit (Innate) and those of Educated (the mind) have different origins, each are transmitted over their special nerves, the splanchnopleure to the inner or visceral portion and the somatopleure to the body wall. These two classes of impulses, destined for different portions of the body, over entirely different divisions of nerves, the one involuntary, the other voluntary, the former devoted to organic life, the latter to animal, ought not be thrown into one indiscriminate lot, as ''Innate mental impulses.''

That Frenchman threw in a question a few evenings ago by saying, although the lady with the head of beautiful flowing hair has a good flow of language, yet there is nothing about her hair that is characteristic of a fluid.

I was referring to physical science, natural philosophy, which deals with the material world. However, any gentle, gradual movement or procedure of thought, diction, or music, which resembles the quiet, steady movement of a river, or a continuous outpouring of words, a stream of language, is referred to as flowing.

It is assumed that all intelligence, our thoughts, every impulse, is formulated in the brain. If so, in what particular part of the brain? Do they originate in the pons, the oblongata, cerebellum or the cerebrum? If in the cerebrum, which half? Is that originating center midway in the corpus callosum, between the two hemispheres? Why not say, I do not know?

In physical science to flow is a type of motion characteristic of fluids, that is, of liquids, gases and viscous solids. A viscous solid is one distinguished by vicosity, having the quality of being adhesive, sticky, ropy or glutinous consistency. Impulses do not flow as a liquid, transudate or circulate as a fluid, or become softened sufficiently to run as a viscous solid. Rivers flow from lakes, tears from the eyes, and the menstrual flow is periodical. Impulses are not liquids, therefore, do not flow. Light heat, sound and impulses are transmitted by vibration—molecular action

—they do not flow. Vital force is inherent, consequently, does not flow.

Impulses are not substances, they are not ponderable, capable of being weighed, they cannot be measured by the bushel, they have no length, breadth or thickness; they do not flow, they cannot be percented, nor impeded, hindered, obstructed or interfered with by the placing of an obstruction in their pathway. The arch or bar of a violin, guitar or other stringed instrument, which gives permanency to and causes the wires or strings to be tensely stretched, do not prevent the passage of vibration. An impingement modifies tension, it changes the amount of vibration, but does not obstruct the course of an impulse; it simply augments or decreases the force of an impulse.

Please remember, abnormal functions and morbid tissue are co-existent.

Howell's Text-Book of Physiology says: "Variations of temperature change the velocity of the impulse, the rate of transmission increases with a rise of temperature up to a certain point. The irritability and conductivity of nerve fibers are influenced markedly by temperature. If a small area of a trunk nerve be cooled or heated the nerve impulse as it passes through this area may be increased or decreased in strength. Impulse conductivity may be entirely suspended by cooling a nerve down to zero, Centigrade; 32 above zero, Fahrenheit. Function promptly returns when the nerves are warmed."

Why are abnormal functions and morbid tissue always associated? Because tissue can only perform functions becoming their condition; structure determines the amount of function. The special action of an organ or other part of the body is determined by the firmness, renitency and tension of tissue.

The truths of biological science have been known for centuries. I made use of them in formulating the science of chiropractic. The principles which compose the science of chiropractic have existed as long as animals have had backbones.

Physicians and surgeons knew of and have taught nerve-tension; neurectasia, nerve-stretching and nerve vibration. They have used, and so have the osteopaths, the stretching of nerves as a therapeutical agent for many years. I was the first to assume that the neuroskeleton was a nerve tension-frame.

Vertebral luxations have been known for many years. I was the first to affirm that slightly luxated joints, those in which the articular surfaces had exceeded their normal limit of movement and there become fixed, was quite common. It was I who first said that about 95 per cent of all diseases were because of luxated joints and that the other five per cent were in other displaced joints.

Many physicians and surgeons have occasionally replaced displaced vertebrae. To D. D. Palmer rightfully belongs the credit of replacing displaced vertebral articulations. See cut on page 220 of The Adjuster.

Before 1895 a few vertebrae were replaced by physicians and surgeons. This was accomplished by main strength and awkwardness. See cut on page 886 of Adjuster.

It has always been held by all practitioners that the blood heated the body in health and disease until July 1, 1903. See cuts on 487 and 489 of the Adjuster.

The different kinds of nerve-pressure have been known to physicians and surgeons. I have added nothing new on pressure. However, I am the first to state that displacements of the joints of the tension-frame cause nerves to become more tense than normal, thereby creating disease.

It has always been held that poisons affected the blood. That bloody delusion will soon be a theorum of the past. Poisons affect nerves. I am the first to say so—what of it. My affirmation will in a measure prevent a lying plagarist from being believed.

I originated nerve-tracing and taught it to my early students while the pseudo fountain head was fishing for tadpoles.

I have succeeded in making displaced articular surfaces adjusting practical. Why not make it definite, specific, scientific?

The Normal and Abnormal Movements of the Vertebral Column.

Muscles or sinews, is one of the contractile organs of the body by which the movements of the various organs and parts are affected. They possess the power of contraction and relaxation. One author says a muscle fibre is from one to five inches in length, another states they vary from a fraction of an inch to many inches. Muscles are directly attached to bones or indirectly by tendons or ligaments, or more definitely speaking they are made fast to the periosteum, the thick fibrous membrane which covers and adheres closely to the entire surface of bones, except, where they are covered with articular cartilge. Muscles in shape may be that of a cord, ribbon or sheet. The surface of bones to which muscles are attached are rough. Laborers have rougher bones than those of clerks. The bones of females are smoother than those of males. Bones become rougher as age advances. Muscles, like nerves, are classed as voluntary and involuntary. The voluntary are those whose actions are under the control of the will; the involuntary control the functions of the internal organs, intestines, blood vessels, etc. The part which is moved by contraction of the muscle is known as the insertion, · or distal, and the fixed or central attachment the origin, or proximal. Skeletal muscles are connected at either or both of their extremities with the bony framework (the tension-frame) of the body. A muscle is attached to two objects; its contraction lessens the distance between them. Motor and sensor nerves end in voluntary muscles. The involuntary muscles are supplied from the sympathetic nerve system. The tendinous portion of a muscle increases with age. The muscles of an adult are stiffer than those of a child, therefore, the range of joint movement is diminished with age, muscular extensibility is greater in youth; as age advances the tendinous inextensibility is increased.

There are three layers of muscles in the back. The superficial, the deep facia and the trapezius. The deep facia is a dense fibrous layer attached to the occipital bone, the spines of the vertebrae, the crest of the ilium and the spine of the scapula. The trapezius muscle is attached to the external occipital protuberance, the spinous process of the seventh cervical and the spinous processes of all the thoracic vertebrae. To the atlas are fastened nine pairs of muscles. To the axis are connected eleven liable to be pinched between the articular surfaces.

Muscles are composed of bundles of reddish fibres, the lean meat of the body, surrounded by a greater or lesser extent by glistening, white connective tissue; they constitute about two-fifths to three-sevenths of

85

the weight of the body. They are known by 230 distinct names. Authors differ as to the number of muscles in the human body, some mention as low as 501, others as high as 682; this difference is accounted for by the anomalous and variable number in different subjects.

A tendon is a nonelastic fibrous cord or band serving to connect a muscle with a bone or other tissue, they are lubricated by synovia.

A ligament is a band or sheet of fibrous, inextensile, pliable, tough and strong tissue connecting the articular extremities of two or more bones, cartilages or other structure, they may serve as supports for fasciae or muscles. Interosseous ligaments with the laminae of the lower 23 movable vertebrae complete the roofing-in of the spinal canal, permit variation in the width of the interlaminar spaces in flexion and extension; they restore the articulating surfaces to their normal position after each movement, and take the place of muscles which would be liable to be pinched between the articular surfacs.

Fasciae covers, ensheaths, supports or binds together internal parts or structures of the body. The word fascia means a band or bandage. Fasciae are divided into superficial and deep. Chiropractors are especially concerned with the deep fasciae which is pearly white, dense, strong, flexible, inelastic, unyielding fibrous membrane, forming sheaths for muscles and affording broad surfaces for attachment. The inner or deep layer of fascia is continuous with the sheaths of nerves, arteries and veins. They not only bind down collectively the muscles, but give a separate cover to each, as well as to blood vessels and nerves. In biology the term fascia is applied to any broad, transverse feathers, hair or scales.

The intervertebral fibrocartilaginous disks are interposed between the adjacent surfaces of the bodies of vertebrae from the axis to the sacrum and between the vertebrae of the sacrum in youth until they become fused; they are the chief bond of connection between these bones. The compressible intervertebral disks constitute pivots round which the bodies of the vertebrae can twist, tilt or incline. The curve of old age is due to the shrinking of the intervertebral substance. The pulp part of these disks form a central elastic pivot or ball, upon and around which the center of the vertebra rests and twists. If it were not for the articular processes which give steadiness to the column the motion would be of a rolling character. There are no fibrocartilaginous disks between the occiput and atlas, nor between the atlas and axis. These rubber-like layers of fibrocartilage are adherent by their surfaces to a thin layer of hyaline cartilage which covers the upper and under surfaces of the bodies of vertebrae.

The intervertebral foramen is formed by the juxtaposition of the upper and lower intervertebral notches or grooves; the upper and anterior portion of which is arranged by the lower border of the pedicle and the posterior lower corner of the body of the superior vertebra. The posterior and lower portion of the foramen is formed by the articular process of the inferior vertebra. The border of the intervertebral foramen is one-fourth smooth and three-fourths rough. There are no muscles, tendons or ligaments attached to the smooth portions of bone. The upper portion of the border of the intervertebral foramen is smooth and the remaining three-fourths roughened for the attachment of ligaments or fasciae. An examination of an intervertebral foramen in the recent state will disclose the trunk of a spinal nerve, which is one-fourth of an inch in length, securely attached by muscles and ligaments to the body of the upper vertebra and the articular process of the lower one adjoining it.

The vertebraterial foramina in the transverse processes of the cervical vertebra form a passage way for the vertebral arteries, veins and plexuses of the sympathetic nerves. This network of nerves surround the arteries and accompany them through the transverse foramina, entering at the sixth and traverse all above it. From the costotransverse foramina of the atlas they enter the skull through the foramen magnum. This interjoining of nerves supply filaments (vasomotor) to the muscle fibres of the arteries and accompany them to the cerebrum and cerebellum. The vertebral plexus communicates by delicate threads with the cervical spinal nerves. The vertebral veins correspond to the extra cranial parts of the vertebral arteries. They form by the union of offsets from the intraspinal venous plexuses, issue from the spinal canal, pass across the posterior arch of the atlas with the vertebral artery to the foramen in the transverse process of the atlas. It then descends through the vertebraterial foramina and breaks up into a plexus of venous channels which surround the artery. These channels unite to form a single trunk which issues from the transverse foramen of the sixth cervical vertebra. Each vertebral vein receives offsets from the intraspinal venus plexus which pass out of the spinal canal by the intervertebral foramina.

The long gap between the occipital bone and the atlas and the intervening space between the atlas and axis are not foramina: no possibility of nerves being pinched, squeezed, occluded, no narrowing of the foramina, no settling in that region. The posterior portion of the ring which surrounds the foramen magnum, the whole surface of the posterior arch of the atlas and the superior of the lamina of the axis are smooth; but few muscles are attached thereunto. There are two distinct sets of articulations in the vertebral column; those between the bodies and intervertebra disks and those between the articular processes.

Arthrodial joints admit of gliding movements: they are formed by the approximation of two plane surfaces, one slightly concave and the other correspondingly convex, the amount of motion between them being limited by ligaments and osseous abutments. The articular surfaces are covered with hyaline cartilage and the bones kept in contact by ligaments.

The transverse ligament of the atlas is a thick, strong band, which arches across the ring of the atlas, and serves to retain the odontoid process in firm connection with the anterior arch. This ligament is flattened from before backward, broader and thicker in the middle than at either extremity, and firmly attached on each side to a small tubercle on the inner surface of the lateral mass of the atlas. This ligament is supplied with a facet, the surface of which is covered with hyaline cartilage. The odontoid process is smaller at the lower part than at the upper portion; it is retained in close connection with the atlas by the transverse ligament embracing tightly its narrow neck.

The vertebral column permits of three distinct movements, gliding, circumduction and rotation. These movements are, however, often, more or less, combined in the various joints and thusly produce quite a variation. It is seldom that we find only one kind of motion in any particular joint.

The movements of the vertebral column are controlled by the shape and position of the articular processes. In the loins the inferior zygapophyses are turned outward and embraced by the superior of its neighbor below; this renders rotation, twisting, of the spinal column in this region impossible. There is nothing to prevent, except, to a certain extent, a sliding movement upward of one and downward of the other, of the two surfaces in contact, known as flexion (bending) and extension (straightening of a curve). In the thoracic region the articulating processes by their direction and mutual adaptation, especially at the upper part of the dorsal series, permit of rotation, but prevent flexion and extension; while in the cervical region the greater obliquity and lateral slant of the articular processes allow not only flexion and extension, but also rotation.

There is only a slight degree of movement between any two individual vertebrae, the atlas and axis excepted, although they permit, as a whole, a considerable change of situation. This slight alteration in the position of the two articular surfaces is allowable, thus far and no farther is normal, a greater separation, or displacement, more than usual, is disease creating. Vertebral displacement is the normal gliding movement exaggerated. The separation of the articular processes increases the distance between the body of the superior vertebra and the articular process of the inferior segment to both of which the spinal nerve trunk is securely moored by stays, known as facise, which are attached to three-fourths of the borders of the foramen; that of the articular process of one vertebra which forms the inferior notch of the foramen, and that of the body of which bounds one-third of the superior notch. Displaced articulations are separated more than usual by oversliding each other, sometimes the separation is complete and accompanied by fracture. The only portions of the vertebral column which permit of being luxated, subluxated, dislocated, displaced are the articular processes. To displace does not mean to crowd together, to shorten the spine by thinning the intervertebral disks or occlude the intervertebral foramina; luxation of the articular processes increase the size of the foramen and the distance between the two places of anchorage of the nerve trunk and its branches, thereby stretching the ligaments and fasciae whereby the trunk of the spinal nerve is secured to three-fourths of the border which is roughened for their attachment, thereby modifying the tension of the nerve trunk and its branches. The above holds true in all intervertebral formania from the axis to the sacrum.

The gliding movement is the most simple kind of motion that can take place in a joint: one surface gliding over another without any angular or rotary movement. This motion is not confined to plane surfaces, but may exist between any two contiguous surfaces, of whatever form, limited by the ligaments which enclose the articulation. An articular displacement increases the separation of the articular surfaces.

Rotation is produced by the twisting of the intervertebral substance (the fibrocartilaginous disks) and a movement between the articular surfaces; this twist and move, although only slight between any two vertebrae, produces a considerable extent of movement when the whole length of the vertebral column is considered. In rotation of the whole vertebral column, the front of the upper part of the spine is turned to one side or the other. There is only one vertebra, the atlas, which really rotates, moves around an axis, the only example furnished in the backbone, the odontoid process serving as a pivot around which the atlas turns. The first and second spinal nerve trunks are anchored to the roughened posterior surfaces above and below the articular processes of the atlas. Any displacement laterally, the only direction in which the atlas can be dislocated, would cause nerves to be stretched, a condition known as nerve tension.

Circumduction is a movement in a circular direction, it is a combination of anterior, posterior and lateral flexion—anterior, posterior and lateral bending.

The normal movement of a vertebral joint may be increased or decreased. Articular displacements, when they remain in a strained position, are disease producers because of creating and continuing nerve tension. Nerve stretching is caused by separating the articular processes, enlarging the foramina, stretching the faciae and other tissue. The intervertebral foramina are not occluded, closed up, narrowed or made smaller. The intervertebral disks are not compressed, made thinner, the nerves are not occluded, pinched or impinged upon. We, as chiropractors, have no use for such unscientific terms as ''The spinal windows are occluded, closed up.''

Forward flexion is a bending of the spine so that the concavity is increased, while the fibres of the opposite side are stretched. The interspace between the laminae of the cervical are widened, and the inferior articular processes of the vertebrae above slide upward upon the articular procsses of the vertebrae below. Flexion is the most extensive of all the movements of the vertebral column. Take your spine in hand, bend it between two vertebrae (the only place it can be flexed) of the dorsal until the articular surfaces are in contact half and half, and you will have created a disease producing displacement, a subluxation, a chiropractic dislocation. The gliding movement of the articular processes can only be performed by extension as each vertebrae of the lower six cervicals and the twelve dorsals are provided with a set of abutments which prevent a downward movement past the normal of the superior articular processes. If such a movement was possible, it would occlude foramina. This gliding movement of the articular surfaces upon each other whether performed in a normal amount or an excess can not do otherwise than enlarge the foramina; this holds true in the lower six cervical, the twelve dorsal and the five lumbar vertebrae. This gliding movement is the most simple kind of motion that can take place in a joint, one surface gliding or moving over another without any angular or rotary movement. This sliding movement is the only one permitted between the articular processes of vertebrae. As I have already said, this gliding movement can only be increased in one direction in the vertebrae named, and such always increases the size of the intervertebral foramina. The two articular surfaces of the articular processes lie face to face in close contact. They are held in this position by pliant, flexible, inextensile, strong, tough ligaments and will not readily yield in any direction except that of the usual gliding movement.

Backward flexion, the movement of the vertebral column backward, an opposite disposition of the parts take place to that of displacement by extension. This movement is very slight, being limited by the imbrication of the laminae and spines, the anterior common ligament, the osseous abutments on the lower six cervical, the twelve dorsal, and lumbar vertebrae. In the dorsal region the close proximity of the spinous processes to each other allow only a very slight extension, backward movement, that which would close the foramina.

In lateral flexion, bending of the body sidewise, the sides of the intervertebral disks are compressed, the extent of motion being limited by the approximation of the transverse processes. This movement may take place in any part of the vertebral column, but has the greatest range in the neck and loins.

The extension movement is a backward flexion, a straightening the spine. This action is limited by the anterior common ligament, the approximation of the spinous processes and the osseous abutments located at the lower edge of the superior articular processes, so that in bending backward the superior processes from the axis to the twelfth dorsal strike against the junction of the transverse processes. The twelfth dorsal is absent of the transverse processes, but more or less supplied with the mammillary processes which serve an admirable purpose for preventing such a movement as would close the foramina. Thus, there is a wise provision throughout the vertebral column to prevent occlusion of the intervertebral foramina.

Flexion and extension are greatest in the lower part of the lumbar region between the third and fourth, and fifth lumbar vertebrae; above the third they are much diminished, and reach their minimum in the middle and upper part of the back. Flexion and extension increase again in the neck, the capability of backward motion from the upright position being in this region greater than that of the motion forward, whereas, in the lumbar region the reverse is the case.

By palpation we determine the spinous process out of alignment because of displacement of the articular processes. Displacing the articular surfaces cause flexion; the bend is shown by the projection of the spinous process above the luxation.

The articulating processes of vertebrae have thin, loose ligamentous sacks, known as capsular ligaments, attached to the margins of their articular surfaces through the greater part of their circumference. They connect the two osseous structures on opposite sides of the intervertebral foramen and hold the blood vessels and nerves in their respective position as they pass through foramina. These thin sheets of pliable tissue are lined on the inner surface with synovial membranes, the function of which is to furnish synovia, a clear, thick, viscid fluid, like the white of an egg, to lubricate the surfaces of these ligaments. The synovial membranes of the vertebral articulations are well supplied with blood vessels and nerves and may become inflamed, known as synovitis. A displacement of the articular surfaces which create the intervertebral foramina, enlarges the size of the aperture, stretches the intervening fasciae, augments nerve vibration of the spinal trunk, causes the filaments to be on a stretch, creates diseased conditions in those parts or organs in which these nerves end. Adjusting, by sliding the articular surfaces back to their normal position, closes the foramen to its normal shape and size, releases undue nerve tension and all is well.

The articulation of the atlas with the axis is of a complicated nature, comprising no fewer than four distinct joints. There is a pivot articulation between the odontoid process of the axis and the ring formed between the anterior arch of the atlas, and the transverse ligament and the posterior of the odontoid. The projection of the axis aids in forming two joints—one in front between the posterior surface of the anterior arch of the atlas and the front of the odontoid process; and another between the anterior surface of the transverse ligament and the back of the tooth-like process. Between the articular processes of the two bones there are double arthrodial or gliding joints in which the opposing surfaces are nearly planes in which there is a gliding motion, which permits the atlas to rotate (and, with it, the cranium) around the projection of the axis, the extent of rotation being limited by the odontoid check ligaments. No rotation can occur between the occiput and atlas. The condyle of the occiput is biconvex, it fits into the biconcave superior articular surface of the atlas. The atlas is the only vertebra which revolves around an axis.

Very rarely the atlas is displaced upward. I saw one specimen which showed plainly two articular surfaces on the front of the odontoid process. I have seen quite a number axeses whose odontoid processes had been extended, lengthened one-sixteenth to one-eighth of an inch by exostosis, a deposit of osseous material upon the apexes of the odontoid processes, evidently for the purpose of preventing the atlas from sliding upward and backward over the tooth-like process.

There is no provision made for a lateral movement of the atlas. Any deviation from the median line, to the left or right, displaces, more or less, four articulations, two of the odontoid process, and two of the articular processes. No one of the four joints can be displaced without a corresponding displacement of all. The odontoid process stands midway between the two tubercles, of the lateral masses, for the attachment of the transverse ligament. These tubercles are in the adult five-eighths of an inch distant from each other. The neck of the odontoid (transverse measurement) is one-fourth of an inch in diameter, leaving a distance of three-sixteenth of an inch on either side of and between the tubercles and the process void of osseous tissue. Occasionally the atlas is displaced laterally to one side or the other, stretching the ligaments, fasciae and nerves which unite the atlas and axis and makes secure not only the spinal cord, but also, the nerves and blood vessels during their passage through the long gaps and emergence from the spinal canal. In all such cases the proper thing to do is to replace the displaced bone, thereby relieve excessive muscl and nerve tension. Between the occiput and axis there are no intervertebral foramina, or intervertebral disks to blame for pinching nerves, abnormal chemical combinations, obstructed currents or occlusion of stimuli.

While the rotary movements are specially arranged for by the peculiar articulations between the atlas and axis, the nodding or rocking motion of the head is permitted by the cups of the superior articular processes and the projecting condyles of the occipital bone. In no one of the skeletal articulations is there a greater diversity in shape and size than in the occipital condyles and their receiving concavities, so much so, that no one condyle can be found to fit in any other than its life-long mate. This variation in size and shape is shown in the condyles and their corresponding articular surfaces of the same occiput and atlas.

In this region I never have had any reason for adjusting, or trying to adjust, the skull or axis, although I have frequent need for replacing the atlas and the third cervical. In adjusting I regard the axis, seventh cervical and sacrum as stationary. A displaced atlas can be easily replaced by giving the thrust against the posterior arch. If the force is thrown against the right half it will spring the anterior arch from the odontoid process sufficient to allow the atlas to move to the left and vice versa.

Vertebrae are occasionally forced out of alignment, the cartilaginous disks torn loose from the bodies. Fractures and osseous ankyloses usually make them immovable; such are surgical displacements of which a chiropractor has nothing to do.

The special features of the above may be verified by anatomical works and dissecting the backbone of human or brute beast.

The movements and displacements of the joints of the foot are of so much concern to chiropractors that I insert a description. A study of their structure, displacements and corrections given by adjusting should relieve us of a lot of absurdities regarding articular displacements which have crept into chiropractic literature.

The skeleton of the foot consists of tarsus, metatarsus and phalanges. The bones of the tarsus are seven in number. Their action is of a slight gliding movement against each other. Like other joints, they are supplied with ligaments, fasciae and synovial membranes. There are no foramina to be sensured for ailments, no intervertebral disks to be thinned by compression. And yet, although the ligaments which hold the tarsal bones together are of great strength, dislocation occasionally occurs. Such displacements cause ''sprained feet''—nerves stretched and inflamed. The portion of the plantar surface in which the nerves end, form calluses and the part of the foot in which the bone is displaced becomes quite painful. By replacing the displaced bone the callus and distress disappears.

The only movements in the phalangeal (toe) joints are flexion and extension. These joints are very liable to be dislocated and calluses appear over or on the sides of the joints known as corns. Those between the toes are called soft corns because of being kept moist. By adjusting the displaced joints the corns will disappear. This may be accomplished at one sitting, or it may take much time, because of illshapened joints and bony or fibrous adhesions.

Medical men can and osteopaths will accept the above facts without due credit—better for the world that is so than not at all. Can you name the chiropractor who will lay claim to being "the developer" of these ideas?

Is it not better to write of what we know, than of that which we know nothing?

A vertebra consists of an anterior solid segment, the body, and a posterior section, the neural arch. The arch is formed of two pedicles, two laminae and seven processes, the two transverse, one spinous and four articular.

The articular processes, four in number, two on either side, each of the two face each other, have a certain amount of movement, which is normal; when this gliding motion becomes increased beyond the normal, it is said to be displaced, dislocated, luxated, the amount depending upon the articular surface exposed. There are two sets of articulations between the movable vertebrae, those between the bodies and those between the articular processes.

Dislocation between two vertebrae (I am speaking of the vertebrae as defined in this article) is almost, if not impossible, such could not occur without a tearing of the intervertebral cartilaginous disks from the bodies of the vertebrae. No chiropractor pretends to replace displaced intervertebral disks. There is no place for a chiropractic displacement, a dislocation, a luxation, except between the articular surfaces of the articulating processes. All vertebrae, except those which deviate from the common vertebral type, present two sets of articulations. The vertebrae are articulated between the centra, known as intercentral, and a pair of articulations between the neural arches called interneural.

The intervertebral disks are located between the verttebral bodies to which they are firmly attached.

The ligaments which unite the component parts of the vertebrae together are so strong, and these bones are so interlocked by the arrangement of their articulating processes, that dislocation of the vertebrae, itself, is very uncommon, unless accompanied by fracture.

Nerves are never pinched or impinged upon in the foramina. Foramina are never narrowed. WE DO NOT ADJUST THE VERTEBRA. The vertebra itself, so far as a chiropractor knows, is never displaced, dislocated or subluxated.

Any extreme movement of the articular surfaces enlarges the foramen or foramina, causes the nerves and blood vessels to become stretched, irritated, increasing its carrying power.

Nerves are never shut off by the closure of the foramina. There are no dams or obstructions that restrict. Impulses are never interrupted.

Reducing the luxated intervertebral articulation; diminishing the displacement of the articular processes, replacing the two articular surfaces, returns the enlarged foramen to its normal size, removes tension and irritation. Irritated nerves cause muscular contraction. The location and amount of disturbance depends upon the portion of the nervous system involved.

A displacement is known by the contour of its angularity, the spinous process will appear to be slightly elevated to the chiropractor who will hold his hand crosswise of the body and run his fingers along the spinal column—not too fast or too slow. Don't do as osteopaths, who run their fingers along on each side of the spinal column to determine what processes are bent to the left or right—these have been foolers to the osteopaths, and chiropractors have dropped into the same rut—don't do anything as an osteopath does. The sliding of the upper surface upward beyond its normal limit causes the spinous process to become more prominent and a slightly greater space will be found between the spinous process of the two vertebrae whose articular surfaces are displaced.

The medical method of reducing a dislocation is, extension, counter extension and coaptation. The chiropractor uses the latter only, the adjusting of two displaced surfaces to each other.

Occasionally one of the spinous processes deviates from the median line, more especially, the center six of the dorsal region, a fact that should be remembered in practice, as they are not significant to a chiropractor, having existed as such since birth and have nothing whatever in common with disease.

Disease is too much or not enough function. About 95 per cent of all diseases are accompanied by slightly displaced articulations—the vertebra is not displaced—the sliding movement of the articulations are increased beyond the normal—consequently, increasing the size of the foramen on one, or the foramina on both sides. The balance of ailments are because of displacement of other joints.

A displacement displaces the articular surfaces, does not crowd, the normal movement is exagerated.

Chiropractors have demonstrated that nerves which innervate certain organs, proceed from one or the other side of the spine. A proven fact: the neuroskeleton is a regulator of tension when its articular surfaces have not been forcibly displaced, separated from their normal bearings, but, articular processes not in normal contact, partially displaced are disease producers.

A surgical luxation has been known to the medical fraternity for centuries, but, a chiropractic luxation was discovered by D. D. Palmer. Chiropractic is unlike any other method or system—don't you forget it.

The ingenuity manifested by chiropractors placing vertebrae in cuts just to suit their fancy is not only amusing but borders upon the ridiculous.

I am making an important distinction between a surgical displacement of vertebrae and a chiropractic dislocation of the intervertebral articular surfaces. I copy a few terms of chiropractors who refer to the vertebrae as defined in this article and by all anatomists. But few chiropractors realize the difference between the two luxations.

In the many cuts of vertebrae I have on hand their abnormal relative position (always made so by hand), the vertebrae are shown as being displaced out of their normal alignment. Judging from the following quotations I am not mistaken in the above statement.

Spinal adjustment. Subluxated spine. Vertebrae depressed. Displaced vertebrae. Vertebral subluxation. Displacement of vertebrae. Vertebrae become displaced. Vertebrae become luxated. Adjusting spinal vertebrae. Adjustment of a vertebra. Vertebrae out of alignment. Partially displaced vertebrae. We adjust displaced vertebrae. Subluxations in the spine. The vertebrae are wrenched, displaced. Chiropractic is the adjustment of vertebrae. Spinal adjustments replace vertebrae into line. Stimulus occluded, normal and abnormal foramina. Vertebral luxations the cause of disease. Shut off the flow of impulses. Do vertebrae stay in place when adjusted? These displacements may be in many directions. Adjustments restore the vertebrae to their normal position. The vertebrae are liable to subluxations or partial displacements. The vertebrae of the spinal are replaced in proper alignment. When vertebrae become luxated, they pinch nerves and they shut off nerve force. It is positively proven that vertebral subluxations are the cause of disease. Cut No. 3 show spines and vertebrae in and out of place. In this cut the lower vertebrae is racked to one side, subluxated, displaced. (Under a cut). Showing how vertebrae can be out of line, pinching nerves. A vertebral subluxation is a mechanical interference with flow of the nerve supply. Between the vertebrae is the only places where the nerves pass between movable bone structures. From subluxations comes the pressure which holds back from the organs and tissues the vitalizing currents. In Cut 1, the second vertebra has been moved backward presenting a partial displacement or subluxation. An accident or strain will cause a displacement or luxation of any one of these vertebrae. A chiropractor with one dextrous thrust adjusts the vertebrae into its natural position, removes the subluxation. In cuts B and D the superior vertebra is luxated (displaced) the spinal openings are occluded (nearly closed).

A prominent writer says: ''The clicking resulting from adjustment can never be shown to be 'that bone has been thrown in place,' as they so strenuously maintain.

''The sudden separation of the facets takes place, and the 'clicking' sound is produced.

''Separating the facets of the two bones—that is the articular surfaces—and lets the air in and gives the sound.''

His Alma Mater taught, ''We find great use for atmospheric pressure to hold bones far enough apart to let the 'joint water' pass freely over the opposing ends of bones.''

Many persons have had the articular surfaces of vertebrae replaced of themselves—accidental chiropractic. These replacements of articular surfaces are accompanied by audible clicks or snaps.

The audible click heard when adjusting is the upper articular process striking against the osseous abutments, the laminae in the lumbar, the shoulders of the laminae in the dorsals, except the 10th, 11th and 12th, which may vary in having the transverse processes broken up into external, superior and inferior tubercules; the superior tubercules answering an admirable purpose of an abutment in preventing the occlusion of the foramina. The atlas strikes against the odontoid process, thereby, causing the audible click.

Spinal Pathogenesis.

Pathogenesis, the generation of disease, the act or process of reproduction, the breeding and production of disease, the origin and genesis of suffering, the development of morbid conditions, or of a diseased character.

Medical men look upon disease as an entity, a something that has an individual living existence, its continuance depending upon its reproduction, therefore, they fight disease, aim to stamp it out; if they could destroy, kill, get rid of every pathogenic germ, the last microbe disease breeder, there would be no such a thing as disease. They consider a disease germ as a special virus, a kind of spore, which by rapid increase causes conditions known as disease, by which disease is communicated. They hold that certain diseases are dependent upon definite micro-organisms. A germ disease is one caused by microorganisms. A microbe is a pathogenic microorganism. They believe that all germ diseases are produced by microbes, that diseases originate from minute microscopic fungi, bacteria, which are developed without or within the body, that unhealthy tissue furnishes food, makes favorable conditions for their rapid multiplication within the animal economy, thereby cause specific diseases which become communicable.

Mental peculiarities, physical characteristics and diseases may be congenital. Congenital is inclusive, it takes in all uterine conditions from concepton to birth. Inborn refers to that whch may be engrafted on the mental or body during development. An infective disease (one which is communicable) may be congenital, not inborn, as are dispositions and constitutional peculiarities which are implanted during development. A physical defect, faulty metabolism, is inborn, a developmental error, acquired during the process of development of the first four months, did not originate because of intrauterine disease or injury.

Chiropractors look upon disease, not as an entity, but a condition in which there is a change in position, structure and functions of organs, that microscopic fungi, or bacteria, are there because of favorable conditions, just as rotting cheese and decaying bread favor the growth of mould. Fungi range in size from the microscopic cells of the yeast plant to the highly organized body of a mushroom.

Drug pathogenesis is the production of morbid symptoms by the use of drugs. A drug is any substance used to return abnormal functionation, or abnormal tissue to normal; any article used as a medicine or in the composition of medicines for external or internal use for the cure of disease.

The history of medicine discloses that each method of treating the

96

sick has been followed by another based on exactly opposite principles and philosophies which are diametrically opposed to each other.

Allopathy. That system of remedial treatment which seeks to cure diseases by producing a condition incompatible with the disease; opposed to homeopathy. "Any poisons must, as Galen held, by counter-poisons be expelled."

Homeopathy. That system of medical treatment which seeks to cure a disease by administering medicine which would produce this same disease in a healthy condition; opposed to Allopathy. Similia similibus curanter. Like cures like.

Spinal pathogenesis includes the origin and development of morbid conditions because of the pathological anatomy of the spine.

In allopathy disease is treated by exciting a morbid (diseased) process of another kind, in another part of the body, a method of substitution.

In Homeopathy, the theory of dynamitization, succussion, trituration, dilution with agitation is said to increase enormously the potency or power of a drug. For example, one part of a crude drug, named salt when used on the table as food, but when it becomes a drug it is sodium chloride. One part of this drug is succussed with nine parts of the sugar of milk. This is known as the first decimal potency. To make the second, one part of the first potency is added to nine parts of sugar of milk, and so on. This trituration may be carried on until there is only one part of salt to a million parts of sugar; this is known as a high potency.

A vertebral column of bones is referred to as a backbone, spinal column and spine. It is not a backbone: it is twenty-six backbones. Taken collectively it is not a spine, although there is a column of spines. It is also called vertebrarium, composed of vertebrae, yet in the whole column there is but one vertebra, the atlas is the only segment which turns (vertere to turn) on a pivot, the ondontoid process. In man the vertebral column is spoken of and understood as being vertical; in quadrupeds horizontal. The twenty-six segments are referred to as a column because they are piled one upon another.

Bony columns are flexuous, having alternate opposite curvatures. They are flexible, capable of being bent without breaking.

The vertebral column supports the head and chest and transmits their weight to the pelvis. It is the axial center of all the movements of the trunk. It lodges and protects the spinal cord, the myelon, spinal marrow, medulla spinalis.

The vertebral notches form foramina, give passage to the vertebral nerves, arteries and veins. The vertebraterial foramina furnish a pathway for the vertebral arteries, veins and the sympathetic plexus of nerves, which innervate the viscera.

Joints are divided into three classes and subdivided into fifteen kinds. The articulations between the bodies of vertebrae form a series of amphiathrodial joints, allowing partial movement in every direction. Those between the articular processes form a succession of arthrodial joints, having a sliding movement.

Upon and within the spinal column are numerous venous plexuses. The veins within the spinal column join those on the outside through the intervertebral foramina.

Pathogenesis is the morbid process, the mode of origin, the development of disease. To learn the cause of disease it is better to examine the living than the dead. To know of and comprehend the position of sublaxated vertebrae, it is preferable to examine vertebral columns which have vertebrae displaced and ankylosed while the owner was living instead of having cuts made of vertebrae ingeneously displaced by hand to suit the fancy.

Pathological means morbid or diseased. A morbid or diseased change in the tissue, bones softened and friable. Morbidity of bones, either too hard, eburnated, or too soft, friable in their texture.

Color, reddish-yellow. Excessive heat has changed the color and consistence of the bones. Bones are formed of white corpuscles, leucocytes. In fever the per cent. of the white and red corpuscles are modified, the red corpuscles, erythrocytes, are increased and the white is diminished. Temperature of 98 to 99 degrees creates the normal, relative number of white and red corpuscles.

Exostosis, a morbid deposit of bone upon the surface of a pre-existing bone. Enostosis, a bony growth on the interior surface of a bone, in the medullary cavity. Hypertrophy, an excessive growth of a part from over-nourishment. Hypoplasia, a lack of development of a bone.

A spinal column before me gives unmistakable evidence of the cause of the morbid condition of those bones. The sixth, seventh and eighth cervicals are ankylosed, spondylosed, the joints immovably fixed by fusion and adhesion. The heat was intense (spondylitis, inflammation of one or more of the vertebrae) that the osseous substance was softened and oozed out, covering the anterior of the bodies of the three vertebrae, ankylosis by fusion. The articular processes are also firmly united, bony union. The displaced sixth cervical is anterior of the normal position, three-sixteenths of an inch out of alignment, causing cervical lordosis. Its transverse processes are anterior of the normal position, thereby stretching the vertebral ganglionic chain which lies in front of and against their anterior surfaces. The intervertebral foramina have not been decreased in size. The whole column shows spondylitis deformans. The luxated vertebra by its pressure against the sympathetic nerve trunk, reaching from the atlas to the coccyx, caused increased nerve tension, liquefaction and fusion, also the same condition in other parts of the vertebral column.

In another backbone I find the ninth, tenth and eleventh dorsal vertebrae ankylosed by fusion of oozed osseous matter, a slight displacement of the ninth dorsal, evidenced by it being slightly tipped laterally, one intervertebral foramen slightly enlarged and the other slightly occluded, the spinous process is depressed anteriorly instead of being elevated posteriorly as usual.

In one other vertebral column a fractured lateral dislocation of the sixth and seventh cervicals. The intervertebral foramina are very much enlarged because of the displacement, the spinous processes widely displaced, no possible chance for the spinal nerves to be pinched. Nerves are impinged upon or against, instead of being pinched between.

The osseous substance of the bodies of the ninth and twelfth dorsal and all the lumbar vertebrae has oozed out and spread upon the bodies of the vertebrae, causing ankyloses by the fusion of liquified bony tissue. Excessive heat caused the softening, lowered the temperature, hardened the callus material.

Several vertebrae are ankylosed by exostoses. Second, third and fourth dorsal vertebrae are ankylosed by fusion of their bodies, the cartilage destroyed by heat.

Formation of scoliotic curvature between second and fourth dorsals.

The ossification of spinalis dorsi muscle renders the contour of the spinous processes as one continuous surface. The spinous processes of the second to the fifth cervical are fractured. The bodies of the cervical vertebrae have been softened by heat and made thin by compression.

The cause of all these morbid conditions is found in the displacement, ankylosis and fracture of the sixth and seventh cervicals; not in the occlusion of the intervertebral foramina for they are enlarged.

The anterior displacement of the sixth cervical, caused the vertebral chain to become tense.

The six cervicals pressed together, show a lordosis, an anterior curvature.

The closure of the vertebraterial foramen, the transverse foramen of the sixth cervical, the elongated pathway for the vertebral artery, vein and the sympathetic plexus of nerves, caused by the displacement, modified nerve tension, vibration and the function of heat.

The spinous processes of second to eighth dorsals curved laterally which was normal to that column.

An ankylosis may be pathological or physiological; fusion may also be pathological or physiological.

The odontoid process was extended to meet the requirement, that of the atlas being displaced upward.

The continuity of local heat throughout the vertebral column transmitted by the ganglionic chains, the vertebral chains, the sympathetic cords, is apparent.

Palpation and Nerve Tracing.

The chiropractor determines the position of bones, more especially those of the vertebral column, the condition and pathway of subdermal nerves, by palpation; this is known as physical diagnosis. This examination is performed by a discriminating touch of the fingers which, directed by knowledge and the skill acquired by continued application, become very sensitive. The truth of the science, the correctness of the art and the reasonableness of its philosophy are demonstrated thereby.

Nerve tracing is an art. The systematic application of knowledge regarding the condition of nerves in health and disease, observation, study, experience and skill acquired by constant practice, has resulted in determining certain principles and facts which enable us to determine the luxated joints, which by their displacement cause more or less nerve-tension, variation of functions, conditions known as disease.

The art of palpation to determine the condition of subcutaneous organs has been used for centuries by medical practitioners. The art of nerve-tracing is of recent date, your teacher was the first to practice it.

The chiropractor should trace sensitive, swollen, longitudially contracted nerves, for the purpose of locating their impingement and tension. By palpation he determines the one or more spinous processes which project posterior of the normal outline. The projection of the displaced spinous process is in the direction of the bend; in the cervical it is anterior, in the dorsal posterior and ventral in the lumbar. In a practice of twenty-five years I have only known one case of reversed kyphosis and lordosis which I relieved by adjusting the twelfth dorsal. There are three vertebrae which may be considered as stationary, the axis, the first dorsal and the sacrum. There is no better way to locate the cause of disease, or demonstrate to a prospective patient how bones and nerves are related to each other and why such relationship accounts for health and disease, than by palpation and nerve-tracing.

By palpation and nerve-tracing the chiropractor can often determine the organ and the innervating subdermal nerves affected. Nerves in their normal condition are not sensitive to pressure; those in the teeth are not affected by cold or hot, sweet or sour ingesta.

By a unique movement the nerve which is unduly stretched, because of being impinged against, or stretched by a displaced bone of the neuro-skeleton, is returned to its normal tension, normal vibration, normal temperature and normal functionating.

Chiropractors demonstrate the correctness of Dr. Dunglison's statement in his dictionary, ''Irritation is indicated by tenderness on pressure over the spinous process of one or more vertebrae or parts of the sides of the spine.''

102

Chiropractors are demonstrating upon living subjects, no cadavers, no vivisection, that there are nerve fibers which have not been noticed by anatomists. Nerve tracing explains this unexplainable explanation of "vicarious commutation," or substitution.

A number of theories have been advanced to explain the process of heredity, the transmission of acquired characteristics, the perpetuation of ancestral distinguishing traits and qualities, including the inheritance of disease from ancestors. One of which is that germinal continuity, minute particles are given off from all cells of the body and collected in the reproductive, generative, living, active basis of all animal organizations; they represent all of the body characteristics, both heredity and acquired.

Medical men believe that the cause of diseases originate outside the body, or are generated within the body. Those outside are, traumatic, heat, cold, poisons and living organisms such as bacteria and animal parasites. Those "originated within the body are less definitely known." "The self-poisoning is designated auto-intoxication."

Pneumonia, diptheria, typhoid fever, measles, mumps, whooping cough and rheumatism are among those diseases acquired by inheritance, transmitted from parent to offspring, physical or mental qualities conveyed from ancestors to their progeny. This theory includes the doubling and multiplication of the vital units of the future individual, which accounts for the variation of form, physical and mental qualities, including the transference of disease. Speculation based on such assumed hypothesis necessarily falls to the ground, as no sharp distinction exists between germ-cells and somatic (pertaining to the wall of the body or the body as a whole) cells.

The above named diseases are classed as those of heredity, whose duration is considered self-limited, are readily relieved by chiropractic adjustments.

Conscious intelligence is the observation of impressions received through the sensory organs of sight, hearing, smell, taste, and touch. To these may be added perception, apprehension, recognition, understanding, discernment and appreciation of our physical surroundings, and these are increased by occult intuition and spiritual instinct, the ability of knowing and the power of acting without the assistance of reason.

Intuitive sense is modified by imagination and memory, by the discriminating qualities of intensification, by the condition of tone and the variation from the standard of health. Modified intuitive sense varies the actions of instinctive consciousness.

Intuitive knowing and instinctive action are determined by organic habits and unconscious sensation without thought or volition.

Instinct is immediate in action without the process of reason.

Intuition consists of knowing without reasoning from cause to effect, direct immediate perception without reasoning.

Instinct is a natural, inherited impulse, unassisted by a reasoning conception of that which occasions or effects a result.

Intuition is the ability of knowing without reason, the immediate perception of truth without conscious investigation, or assigning rational causes for their existence.

Instinct is an inward unconscious principle in man and the lower animals, an involuntary prompting which causes mental or physical action without individual experience or a distinct apprehension of the end to be accomplished, an innate tendency to perform a special action in a distinctive way when the necessity occurs.

Intuitive belief, intuitive judgment and intuitive knowledge are qualities due to direct perception, the result of inward consciousness. Intuition may be mystical, perceptional, intellectual or moral. We may have mystical vision, spiritual perception and direct intellectual apprehension.

Hexiology is the science of habits. A habit is a tendency to perform the same spontaneous action under similar circumstances. Habit applies to individuals, instinct to ancestors. Habits acquired through our ancestors are known as instinct.

Organic habits may be acquired by the physical organism during the life of an individual or of a race. The system of bodily processes of the physiological organism has been acquired through past generations.

Constant practice, frequent repetition, habitual custom, confirms habit until it becomes a function. Mental or organic habits are acquired through the education of the nervous system.

In biology our environments are the aggregate of all the external conditions and influences affecting the life and development of an organism. In a measure we regulate our surroundings, giving but little thought of individual and organic habits. Pernicious habits may become fastened upon the human will, weaken vitality and bore tunnels through the reservoirs of force and character. Self-respect and restraint of passions are as essential to longevity as prophylaxis, the science and art of retaining the health. Desides that are dangerous must be shunned; the mind must be kept wholesome.

Every time we think, each time we act, a record is made. Each repetition of a thought, each performance of an act deepens the groove of habit, mental or physical; it renders the next similar impulse or movement more automatic until in time the nervous system becomes like a phonograph disk; without apparent consciousness we find ourselves guilty of repetition. Habits become our master and we its slave.

Pure air, clean water, unadulterated food and thoughts free from error and vulgarism will form cleanly habits of mind and body.

Chiropractors should comprehend the principle of reflex action.

Reflex is the bounding back, the return of an impulse. A reflex action is one executed without our will, one performed and directed by that intelligence which controls the sympathetic nervous system, the nerves of organic life. An involuntary movement of an organ or part of the body resulting from an impression carried by a sensory or afferent to a subordinate center, and then sent back by an efferent nerve to some place at or near the source of irritation is known as reflex action.

All acts performed without brain function are known as reflex actions. The involuntary brushing a fly from the face, or the attempt to move away from an annoyance when tickled with a feather are examples. In reflex acts, a person does not think before he acts; he acts before he thinks. The nervous impulse comes from the outside and returned, is acted upon without going to the cerebrum. As it were, the message is short-circuited back to the surface by motor nerves, without having reached the thinking centers. Automatic acts are accomplished without thinking. By training the acts have become automatic. Habits are really acquired reflex actions. Habit trains certain nerve centers.

Reflex action is the bounding back of an impulse; the conveyance of an impression from the central system, and its transmission back to the periphery through a motor nerve. The amount of function depends upon the renitency, the impulsive force obtained by the bounding back, the reflex action.

A reflex pathway is the route taken by an impulse; it includes the afferent nerve, the nerve-center and the efferent nerve.

A reflex center is any ganglionic center where a sensory impression is changed into a motor impulse.

Sneezing and the involuntary sniffing of an odor, whether pleasant or unpleasant, are reflex actions. Coughing and choking may be produced by tickling the pharynx, reflex actions, the performance of functions by the controlling intelligence without using the encephalon. Accumulated urine and feces call for micturition and defecation, reflex action.

An enlarged, contracted, sensitive nerve may in reality be only a nerve fiber which may leave a nerve (a bundle of fibers) and enter another; thus, we trace many nerve fibers from their exit at the spinal foramen to their destination, or vice versa, nerve filaments which have not been recognized by anatomists.

Be careful to make a distinction between palpation, perceiving by the sense of touch and palpitation, rapid pulsation of the heart.

Bones and Nerves.

Medical, osteopathic and chiropractic schools give more or less attention to the study of osteology and neurology, but not a page, paragraph or even a sentence is found in any one of the many works I have on anatomy, neurology, physiology and pathology regarding the all important fact that, the position of bones has all to do with the amount of nerve tension.

Dr. A. P. Still's philosophy and mechanical principles of osteopathy, "date 1902," has less than a half page referring to the vertebral column. He says, "Every joint of the neck and spine has much to do with a healthy heart and lungs, because all vital fluids pass through the heart and lungs.

"He (the osteopath) should . . . never rest day or night until he knows the spine is true and in line from atlas to sacrum, with all the ribs in perfect union with the processes of the spine.

"Slipped or twisted vertebrae and ribs must be sought out and adjusted, giving intercostal nerves thorough freedom to act and soften muscles and let blood loose to feed and nourish the whole spine.

"Adjust the bones of the neck and let blood flow to and feed the nerves and muscles of the neck and stop the constrictures that have been holding the blood in check until it has died."

Doctor Still, the founder of osteopathy, believed that wind, air, electricity and gas existed in the joints, between the articular surfaces, that a change in the amount of these fluids accounted for health and disease. I quote from page 130. "Before pain begins at the joints you are sure to find that all gas or wind has left the joints. Thus, electricity burns because of bone friction. Some gas must be between all bone joints. Thus, we find great use for atmospheric pressure to hold bones far enough apart to let the joint water pass freely over the opposing ends of bones. There is a natural demand for gas in all healthy joints of the body. Reason leads us to believe that gas is constantly being conveyed to or generated in all joints. Before rheumatism appears the separating gas has been exhausted, and there follows friction and electric heat because of there being two or more joints in one electric current or division.

"We thus get what we call neuralgia, rheumatism, sciatica, and so on to the full list of aches and pains not accounted for to date by our philosophers.

"On this plane of reason you can see and know the whys of consumption, dropsy, tumors, fits, grey hair, baldness, and so on to a surprising number of diseases."

The above does not read like, nor is its philosophy that of chiropractic. Evidently, Dr. Still was looking to joints for the cause of
disease.

On the title page of McClelland's Regional Anatomy, two large
volumes, Date 1892, is a line in French, in English it says, ''Anatomy is
not such as is taught in schools.'' In other words, anatomy as taught
in schools is not anatomy.

Schools of chiropractic put in many months studying anatomy. The
students are led to believe that the study of anatomy furnishes the all
important education for a chiropractor, that to know anatomy is to
understand chiropractic. A course in dissecting and the different branches
of medicine will not furnish the principles of chiropractic, reason out its
philosophy, nor educate one in vertebral adjusting.

Bones give rigidity and shape to the body, form a case around the
brain and spinal cord, protect delicate organs in the body cavities, constitute a frame-work of which individual bones are used as levers by
muscles and nerves. In many invertebrate animals the muscles are attached to the exoskeleton. In man they are connected to the endoskel-
eton. Bones serve as a tension-frame; their position determines the
amount of muscle and nerve tension. Nearly half of the body weight
is of muscle. Movements are performed by means of muscles, leverage
is obtained by their attachment to bones. Displaced bones cause muscles
and nerves to become stretched or relaxed.

Traumatism is a diseased condition of the system due to an injury
or a wound.

Luxated joints, more especially those of the vertebral column, cause
traumatism, a diseased condition. Dislocated bones impinge upon nerves,
cause irritation; or, by their displacement relax or elongate the nervous
tissue, thereby modifying tension, vibration, the transmission of impulses,
the production of heat and organic function.

Poisons affect nerves, cause their relaxation or contraction. Loss of
tension produces atony, enervation, a diminution of muscular power.
Innervation is increased by nerve contraction. Contracted nerves by
their action on muscles draw vertebrae out of alignment.

Autosuggestion, or hypnotism (suggestion by another) relaxes or
contracts nerve tissue, causing more or less tension.

The importance of bone pressure, nerve impingement, nerve tension,
the all important fact that the position of the osseous frame, the neuroskeleton of the human body, has all to do with the amount of nerve
tension, normal or abnormal, known as nerve strain, the amount of heat,
is never mentioned, in fact, is never thought of by the teachers of medical
or chiropractic schools. It is, therefore, manifest that, the would-be
teachers of chiropractic know but little of the principles of chiropractic,
do not know of it as a science, or of its philosophy.

Nerve tension is accomplished by the bones acting as levers. A knowledge of this principle is essential for the comprehension of chiropractic as a science, and specific adjusting as an art.

A student may become familiar with the different branches of anatomy by the study of one or more books and dissection on the cadaver, and yet not know anything of the relationship existing between bones and nerves. Knowing the structure of bones and nerves, the names of each and all their surfaces, the descriptive terms, nomenclature and classification, their location and functions, do not inform us of the importance which chiropractors should attach to the position of bones.

Do not forget for one moment that, all vital and intellectual forces depend upon the condition of the nervous system for their expression, that there is a vital principle which distinguishes organized matter from inorganic, that when associated with matter of organized bodies controls its manifestation.

Bones are the only hard substances which can press against, impinge upon nerves, by their displacement cause nerves to become stretched. Displaced bones are the direct cause of a large per cent. of diseases. Any pressure upon or against nerves excites and creates abnormal tension. Bones displaced ever so little cause nerves to become contracted or relaxed; either condition modifies vibration, alters the force of an impulse and the amount of heat.

A knowledge of the structure of bones and nerves is well and good. To be able to name and locate the depressions, articular and nonarticular eminences is of especial benefit to surgeons, but to a chiropractor it is all important and of more service to be acquainted with the relationship existing between bones and nerves. In order to have health, nerves must have normal tension, innervate each and every organ of the body, so that their functions may be properly performed.

Displaced bones, luxated or fractured, cause disease (not ease), by overtension of nerves, therefore, chiropractors should be especially interested in the study of bones and nerves, more particularly regarding the effect either one has upon the other.

See pages 761 and 766 of The Adjuster.

Normal nerve tension depends upon the usual position of bones. Displaced bones modify nerve tension, vary the amount of heat. Molecular vibration produces heat in animate and inanimate bodies. Excessive nerve vibration, molecular disturbance, causes inflammation. Diffused inflammation is known as fever; heat expanded, spread, scattered, extended, dispersed throughout the body is known as fever.

Pyorrhea Alveolaris.

Pyorrhea alveolaris has been extensively written upon by Fauchard, Riggs and many others; it is known as Fauchard's disease, also Riggs' disease.

Alveolar pyorrhea is an oozing of pus from beneath the gum margins; a resorption of the alveolar borders, with progressive loosening of the affected teeth, and a deposition of calcic matter, calcium, lime, known as calculi, upon the surface of the denuded roots. With the loss of teeth these morbid conditions cease. It is a disease of adult life, seldom found before the age of thirty years, owing to the pliability of nerve tissue during youth. Nerve tissue becomes firmer, less elastic, as age advances, therefore it does not so readily adapt itself to heat modifications. Pus is composed of leucocytes, white corpuscles. The proportion of white and red corpuscles varies slightly in different persons in health, in various portions of the body and at different ages in the same individual, owing to slight deviations of temperature; the normal amount is one of white to 700 of red. In fever the per cent of erythrocytes is increased. When the temperature goes below 98 degrees the proportion of leucocytes is increased. **Alveolaria** is pertaining to the alveoli. The alveola is the socket in which the tooth rests. **Pyorrhea alveolaris** refers to a discharge of pus from the opening in which the tooth is held. **Pyorrhea** is a disease of the dento-alveolar joint, a gomphosis articulation, one in which a conic process is held in place by a socket, which permits a certain degree of motion. Extraction of the teeth puts an end to the disease by eliminating this membranous joint; it removes, with the teeth, the intervening pericementum. An inflammation of this membrane is known as **pericementitis. Alveolitis** is an inflammation of the alveoli, the bone surrounding the roots of the teeth; the alveoli become necrosed because of too much heat. **Alveolar periostitis** is an inflammation of the alveola periosteum. The periosteum is a thin vascular membrane of the alveoli, closely adhered to and covering the outer surface of the pericementum. The function of the periosteum is to nourish the alveoli by vasa vasorum. This vascular circulation is controlled by and thru the nervi vasorum. Osteo-periostitis is an inflammation of the bone and its periosteum. **Interstitial gingivitis** is an inflammation of the gums, more especially the tissue between the gum and the teeth. The teeth become loose the gums red and swollen and sensitive. The gums are composed of dense fibrous tissue covered by mucous membrane, are richly supplied with blood vessels, but sparsely with nerves. Around the neck of the teeth, at the gingival, the gum forms a free overlapping collar, the dental ligament, where it is freely supplied with nervous papilla, visible to the naked eye. **Cementoperiostosis** is an inflammatory condition of the cementum of the teeth. Cementum is the outer cortical substance, the substantia ossea, the crusta petrosa, the rocky crust, a form of modified bone, which covers the roots of the teeth and answers a similar purpose as does the periosteum of the alveoli. The alveoli-dental pericementum, peridental membrane, or root membrane, is a vascular layer of connective tissue attached to and lying between the periosteum of the walls of the alveoli and the cementum of the roots of the teeth. When the pericementum, which is well supplied with blood vessels and nerves, is inflamed, it becomes swollen and very sensitive. The tooth, as a result of the swelling, is pushed partly out of its socket, its crown projects above those of its neighbors, and strikes against the opposite tooth, causing pain and much annoyance. The alveolar periosteum is firmly united to the root cementum by perforating fibers, establishing a communication of blood vessels and nerves between the jaw and the teeth. **Pericementitis** is an inflammatory condition of the peridental membrane. The pericementum, the interstructural membrane, is composed of white fibrous tissue, interlaced with blood vessels, nerves and glands; it is, therefore, liable to be inflamed, as other membranous tissue. It subserves the purpose of a ligament, similar as the pericranium performs in the sutures of the cranial bones. The same blood vessels and nerves supply the periosteum, pericementum and cementum. **Periostitis**, gingivarium, is an inflammation of the gums and their surroundings. **Ulitis** is an inflammation of the gums. **Gingivitis expulsiva** is the gradual loosening and expulsion of a tooth or teeth from their sockets.

The teeth are composed of four specialized tissues—enamel, dentine, crusta petrosa and the pulp. Between the root of the tooth and the alveolar process are the cementum and the periosteum, interposed between the latter two membranes is the pericementum. The roots of the teeth have small apertures in their apices, which transmit blood vessels and nerves to the pulp cavity, which is filled with pulp. The sockets of the alveoli are lined with periosteum, covering them closely, and intimately uniting the cementum with the fibrous structure of the gums.

The pathological condition of cementoperiostosis is slow progressive expulsion of the teeth. If the M. D.'s had this disease to treat they would class it among the incurable—etiology obscure. Some dental authors ascribe decayed teeth as the cause, altho they know that the most of teeth so expelled are perfectly sound. Were they correct in their etiology of this cementoperiostitic condition that periodontitis is caused by any one of the fifteen lesions given by dental authors, it would be an unexplainable explanation, for we would want to know the cause of dental caries.

Pyorrhea and dental necrosis should be classed as two separate conditions, two different nerves impinged upon, creating two distinctly different morbid conditions of tissue and dissimilar abnormal functions.

The dental profession has made much study of this disease known by several names. They have no trouble in designating the parts affected; the morbid conditions and symptoms are readily apparent. They are well acquainted with the pathological functions and morbid tissue, but as to the cause of the morbid changes in and around the alveoli, they are unable to give us any light thereon. Its etiology remains obscure. Many, very many, remedies have been tried in vain.

The body is composed of myriads of cells; the teeth and their surroundings are no exception. These have the quality of form alteration; they possess the ability to contract and expand, known as latent energy. This energy is controlled and modified by heat; the amount of heat is determined by nerve-vibration, heat being a function of nerves. Extremes of temperature, above or below normal, softens or hardens tissue, induces necrosis or sclerosis. A living organism, or any of its organs, possess a certain degree of action and function, a condition when normal known as health. When functions are raised or lowered from the general average, a condition of disease exists. Nerve irritation increases temperature. Cell metabolism is a heat production. Energy is stored in the cells of organs as a latent agent ready to be used as a functional force directed by impulses. Extremes of heat and cold induce the various phases of inflammation by contracting nerve tissue longitudinally. Heat within certain defined limits is essential to the development of all organized beings. Excessive heat when applied to tissue, external or internal, causes its expansion, converts it from the solid into the fluid state. Any interference with the normal response of an impulse results in morbid physiology—pathology.

All functions in any degree are controlled by and dependent upon nerve impulses. Fear causes a contraction of the blood vessels of the head and face; shame and anger a dilation of the same vessels; these two conditions are the result of nervi vasorum force on the vaso vasorum. With the cessation or the disappearance of the emotional state, the blood vessels return to their former degree of contraction. The flushed condition shown by redness and excessive heat is the result of an accumulation of blood in the capillaries. The whitened, colorless, pallid cuticle is from a lack of ordinary nerve vibration; undulation is dependent upon excitation of nerves.

Alveola pyorrhea is always associated with nephritis, an inflammatory condition of the kidneys. For many years I observed that every patient having pyorrhea of the gums had Bright's disease, but not

every one affected with nephritis has alveolar pyorrhea. Fibers of
the twelfth pair of dorsal nerves go to and innervate the kidneys,
gums and eyelids.

Inflammatory disturbances involve an interstitial gingivitis, an infiltration of leucocytes into the interstices of connective tissue of the
gum. When inflammation is confined to the margin of the gums
adjoining the necks of the teeth, it is specialized as marginal gingivitis.
The effect of a low-grade inflammation is the ossifying or resorption
of the cementum, substantia ossea dentium, the crust of osseous substance covering the roots of the teeth or periosteum of the bones.

The alveolar process is that portion of the maxillary bone which
surrounds and supports the tooth. The surface of bone lining the
alveolus is pierced by many passages for blood vessels which furnish
nutriment to the pericementum and cementum. These contain in the
musculature a plexus of vaso-motor nerves, vasoconstrictors and vaso-
dilators, which control dilation of the blood vessels. In the physio-
logic condition these fibers are in a state of continual contraction,
giving to the arteries and veins a certain average caliber which not
only permits, but by normal impulsive force causes a definite volume
of blood to flow thru them in a given unit of time. The tonic contraction and expansion, diastole and systole, is due to and modified
by the amount of heat, a result of nerve vibration. The tonicity of
the vacsular muscles is subject to increase or decrease in accordance
to the quantity of nerve vibration and heat production; these are
always correspondent in their amounts. Increased contraction results
in a decrease of diameter of blood vessels and a reduction in the out-
flow of the blood. The small arteries thus determine the volume of
blood passing to any given area or organ in accordance with its functional activities. The vaso-motor nerves pass directly from the spinal
nerves to the muscle-fibre through the inseparable, vibratory nerve-
movement and the resultant heat therefrom, the internal diameter
of the blood vessels and the volume of the blood are accurately adapted
to the needs of each organ. During the rest and activity the blood
vessels and nerves maintain a constant tone, normal renitency, elasticity, activity, strength and excitability, as observed in a state of
health.

The nerves of the pericementum are derived from the fifth cranial
or trigeminal nerve and the sympathetic nervous system; they enter
by the apical tissue and the alveolar wall.

Lippincott says, Exostosis (hypercementosis), pyorrhea alveolaria,
necrosis of the jaw (alveolar cancer), recession of the gums, stomatitis
(inflammation of the mouth), gingivitis and gum boils, are due to inflammation of the tissues around the teeth.

It is true, all of these morbid conditions are attended by inflammation, are the result of excessive heat. Chiropractically, these diseases should be placed in three clases: Pyorrhea, recession of the gums; gingivalgia, pain in the gums, and gingivitis, inflammation of the gums. Gingivalgia, pain in the gums, and gingivitis, inflammation of the gums, are because of an impingement on the twelfth pair of dorsal nerves, while hypercementosis, caries of the teeth, alveolar burrowing abscesses, toothache and gum boils are due to an impingement on the third pair of cervical nerves. Stomatitis can be relieved by removing pressure from off the right fifth dorsal nerve.

The dental profession give as probable causes of gingivitis that of uric acid diathesis, mercurial poisoning, gonorrheal infection, bacteria, drug action, faulty metabolism, auto-intoxication, irritants in the blood and distu. bed peripheral nutrition, as systemic causes; that of malocclusion, overuse and disuse of the teeth, as mechanical excitants, and a lack of, or an excess of, friction, and fermentable material lodged about the necks of the teeth, as local causes.

I discovered and have proven by relieving a number of cases that expulsive gingivitis is caused by inflammation of the twelfth pair of dorsal nerves, a portion of the fibers of which ramify the gums as nervi vasorum. A relief of this nervous affection may be had by removing the impingement on these nerves.

Burchard's Dental Pathology states: "In cases of hypercementosis it is assumed that the source of irritation is pressure upon the nerves of the pericementum by the hypertrophic growth. Very widespread disorders may arise from this source."

Burchard assumes that widespread disorders (spreading over many and varied conditions of disease) of the teeth and gums may arise from pressure upon nerves. Chiropractors do not, or, at least should not, assume the source of irritation. They should know the origin of disease, and be scientific as well as efficient in the art of adjusting.

Burchard mentions trifacial neuralgia as being a reflex disturbance from pressure upon nerves. Trifacial neuralgia includes odontalgia, toothache and neuralgia maxillaris.

A reflex action is one executed without consciousness. Such movements are accounted for by chiropractors as a bounding back—a return of an impulse—a motor, impulsive response to a sensory impulse—the conveyance of an impression to the central nervous system and its transmission thru a motor nerve to the periphery. A reflex or reflected pain, according to pathologists, is one referred to some location other than that of its origin. This definition, if accepted by chiropractors, would define all pains as being reflex, originating in one locality by an impingement on a nerve, and its expression of disease, in another area, at its peripheral ending.

Dental neuralgia, odontalgia, toothache and dental caries arise from nerve excitation of the third pair of cervical nerves, the cause of inflammatory conditions, while that of the hard tissue of the gums because of pressure on the twelfth pair of dorsal nerves, the cause of dental neuralgia and caries, can be traced to the third pair of cervical nerves.

Through the intestinal sympathetic connection of the fifth cranial nerve with the seventh, ninth and tenth cranial nerves, salivary, muscular, nervous, alimentary and pulmonary disturbances become possible.

Pathological dentition readily demonstrates the relationship existing between pressure-impingement, irritation, inflammation and their "reflex disturbances." Increased dental temperature stimulates the salivary glands, increases the flow of saliva, creates a disturbance of functional activity—functions performed in excess is disease.

Fever is diffused inflammation. Temperature above that of normal creates disease. Impulsive nerve-vibration determines the amount of heat. The degree of heat of the body of a living being regulates the amount of function. Functions performed above or below normal creates conditions known as disease.

Burchard affirms: "Neuralgia pain is a condition produced thru the overexcitation of any portion of a sensory nerve. The causes should be sought for and, if possible, removed." Chiropractors are able to locate the cause of nerve overexcitation and relieve toothache in less than a minute by the removal of pressure.

Burchard tells us that overuse, abuse and disuse of the teeth are causes which produce inflammation of the pericementum (interstitial gingivitis), inflammation of the gums, resulting in purulent or non-purulent liquefaction (necrosis) of the gingival (gum) portion of the pericementum (pyorrhea alveolaris).

Burchard blames dental irritation for gout, obstinate pains in the toes and fingers, also sciatica, ovarian and uterine neuralgia. He speaks of violent attacks of trifacial neuralgia as a common reflex disturbance from functional disorders of the eye and ear, and motor disturbances of chorea, epilepsy, paralysis, malaria, syphilis and amenia as producing neuralgia. The same old Allopathic explanation—one disease produces another. He fails to grasp the fact of nerve-distribution, that a nerve is composed of one or more fibers, which ramify one or more areas, consequently one or more affections, in as many parts of the body, may arise from one impingement upon a nerve containing many fibers. He maintains that neuralgia pains in the teeth are because of pressure on exposed dentine, that pulp degeneration as a cause of affections outnumber all others.

Dentists and physicians are alike in ascribing one disease as the cause of another, and, that other is the cause of the one, simply from the fact that two or more affections are frequently associated together. Chiropractors elucidate this heretofore mysterious connection of morbid anatomy and functional variation of two or more organs, collectively known as disease.

CPSIA information can be obtained
at www.ICGtesting.com
Printed in the USA
LVOW06s1603210717
541863LV00010B/260/P